Medicine

PreTest®
Self-Assessment
and Review

· NOTICE ·

Medicine is an ever-changing science. As new research and clinical experience broaden our knowledge, changes in treatment and drug therapy are required. The editors and the publisher of this work have checked with sources believed to be reliable in their efforts to provide information that is complete and generally in accord with the standards accepted at the time of publication. However, in view of the possibility of human error or changes in medical sciences, neither the editor, nor the publisher, nor any other party who has been involved in the preparation or publication of this work warrants that the information contained herein is in every respect accurate or complete and they are not responsible for any errors or omissions or for the results obtained from use of such information. Readers are encouraged to confirm the information contained herein with other sources. For example and in particular, readers are advised to check the product information sheet included in the package of each drug they plan to administer to be certain that the information contained in this book is accurate and that changes have not been made in the recommended dose or in the contraindications for administration. This recommendation is of particular importance in connection with new or infrequently used drugs.

Medicine

PreTest®
Self-Assessment
and Review

Sixth Edition

Edited By

Mark I. Taragin, M.D., M.P.H.
Assistant Professor of Medicine
Department of Medicine, Division of General Internal Medicine
University of Medicine and Dentistry of New Jersey—
  Robert Wood Johnson Medical School
New Brunswick, New Jersey

McGraw-Hill, Inc.
Health Professions Division/PreTest® Series
New York   St. Louis   San Francisco   Auckland
Bogotá   Caracas   Lisbon   London   Madrid
Mexico   Milan   Montreal   New Delhi   Paris
San Juan   Singapore   Sydney   Tokyo   Toronto

Medicine: PreTest® Self-Assessment and Review

6 7 8 9 0   DOCDOC   9 8 7 6 5 4 3

ISBN 0-07-051989-7

The editors were Gail Gavert and Bruce MacGregor.
The production supervisor was Clara B. Stanley.
R.R. Donnelley & Sons was printer and binder.
This book was set in Times Roman by R.J. Landi Book Production.

Library of Congress Cataloging-in-Publication Data

Medicine : PreTest self-assessment and review -- 6th ed. / edited by
  Mark I. Taragin.
      p.   cm.
  Includes bibliographical references.
  ISBN 0-07-051989-7
  1. Medicine -- Examinations, questions, etc.   2. National Board of
Medical Examiners -- Examinations -- Study guides.   3. Federation of
State Medical Boards of the United States -- Examinations -- Study
guides.   4. Educational Commission for Foreign Medical Graduates -
- Examinations -- Study guides.   I. Taragin, Mark I.
  [DNLM: 1. Medicine -- examination questions. W 18 M4914]
R834.5.M4   1991
616'.0076 -- dc20
DNLM/DLC
for Library of Congress   90-13705
                                                                    CIP

Contents

Contributors *vii*

Preface *ix*

Introduction *xi*

Allergy and Immunology
Questions *1*
Answers, Explanations, and References *10*

Infectious Disease
Questions *21*
Answers, Explanations, and References *32*

Rheumatology
Questions *44*
Answers, Explanations, and References *51*

Pulmonary Disease
Questions *62*
Answers, Explanations, and References *69*

Cardiology
Questions *78*
Answers, Explanations, and References *93*

Endocrinology and Metabolic Disease
Questions *109*
Answers, Explanations, and References *122*

Gastroenterology
Questions *138*
Answers, Explanations, and References *145*

Nephrology
Questions *153*
Answers, Explanations, and References *159*

Oncology and Hematology
Questions 167
Answers, Explanations, and References 177

Neurology
Questions 188
Answers, Explanations, and References 196

Dermatology
Questions 206
Answers, Explanations, and References 212

Bibliography *219*

Contributors

Louis F. Amorosa, M.D.

*Associate Professor of Clinical Medicine
Department of Medicine, Division of
Endocrinology
UMDNJ—Robert Wood Johnson Medical
School
New Brunswick, New Jersey*

Jerry M. Belsh, M.D.

*Associate Professor of Clinical Neurology
Department of Neurology
UMDNJ—Robert Wood Johnson Medical
School
New Brunswick, New Jersey*

Richard M. Berger, M.D.

*Clinical Professor of Medicine
Department of Medicine, Division of
Dermatology
UMDNJ—Robert Wood Johnson Medical
School
New Brunswick, New Jersey*

Mitchell S. Cappell, M.D., Ph.D.

*Assistant Professor of Medicine and
Director, Gastrointestinal Motility and
Laser Endoscopy Unit
Department of Medicine, Division of
Gastroenterology
UMDNJ—Robert Wood Johnson Medical
School
New Brunswick, New Jersey*

Perry Cook, M.D.

*Assistant Professor of Medicine and
Director, Lymphoma Service
Department of Medicine, Division of
Neoplastic Diseases
New York Medical College
Valhalla, New York*

Douglas Hutt, M.D.

*Assistant Professor of Medicine
Department of Medicine, Division of
Pulmonary and Critical Care
UMDNJ—Robert Wood Johnson Medical
School
New Brunswick, New Jersey*

Clifton R. Lacy, M.D.

*Assistant Professor of Medicine
Department of Medicine, Division of
Cardiovascular Disease and
Hypertension
UMDNJ—Robert Wood Johnson Medical
School
New Brunswick, New Jersey*

Catherine A. Monteleone, M.D.

*Assistant Professor of Medicine
Department of Medicine, Division of
Allergy, Immunology, and Infectious
Diseases
UMDNJ—Robert Wood Johnson Medical
School
New Brunswick, New Jersey*

Leonard Sigal, M.D.

*Associate Professor, Departments of
Medicine and Molecular Genetics and
Microbiology
Department of Medicine, Division of
Rheumatology
UMDNJ—Robert Wood Johnson Medical
School
New Brunswick, New Jersey*

Ajay Singh, M.D.

*Assistant Professor of Medicine
Department of Medicine, Division of
Nephrology
UMDNJ—Robert Wood Johnson Medical
School
New Brunswick, New Jersey*

Steven J. Sperber, M.D.

*Assistant Professor of Medicine
Department of Medicine, Division of
Allergy, Immunology, and Infectious
Diseases
UMDNJ—Robert Wood Johnson Medical
School
New Brunswick, New Jersey*

John Walker, M.D.

*Associate Professor of Clinical Medicine
Department of Medicine, Division of
Nephrology
UMDNJ—Robert Wood Johnson Medical
School
New Brunswick, New Jersey*

Preface

A physician is entrusted with an awesome responsibility—human life. This commitment is rewarded by the satisfaction of assisting people through difficult circumstances and the fulfillment of developing long-term relationships. To effectively meet this obligation, and maintain expertise, requires extensive training built upon a strong foundation of knowledge.

Much has transpired in this ever-changing, exciting field of medicine. Therefore, this edition has been extensively revised by the contributing editors, experts in their respective fields. Not only are they outstanding clinicians, they are also academicians with an awareness of recent developments. They have made significant changes throughout this text, and many sections have been totally rewritten. I thank them for a job well done. Additionally, I encourage you to provide us with comments and suggestions to improve this text in the future.

This book should provide you with a useful self-assessment of your proficiency while simultaneously expanding your fund of knowledge. May your quest for wisdom be never-ending, yet fulfilling.

Mark I. Taragin, M.D., M.P.H.

Introduction

Medicine: PreTest® Self-Assessment and Review, 6th Ed., has been designed to provide medical students, as well as physicians, with a comprehensive and convenient instrument for self-assessment and review within the field of medicine. The 500 questions provided have been designed to parallel the format and degree of difficulty of the questions contained in the Comprehensive Part II of the National Board of Medical Examiners examinations, the Federation Licensing Examination (FLEX), and the Foreign Medical Graduate Examination in the Medical Sciences (FMGEMS). This book will continue to be a useful study tool for Step 2 of the United States Medical Licensing Examination (USMLE).

Each question in the book is accompanied by an answer, a paragraph explanation, and a specific page reference to either a current journal article, a textbook, or both. A bibliography that lists all the sources used in the book follows the last chapter.

Perhaps the most effective way to use this book is to allow yourself one minute to answer each question in a given chapter; as you proceed, indicate your answer beside each question. By following this suggestion, you will be approximating the time limits imposed by the board examinations previously mentioned.

When you have finished answering the questions in a chapter, you should then spend as much time as you need verifying your answers and carefully reading the explanations. Although you should pay special attention to the explanations for the questions you answered incorrectly, you should read every explanation. The authors of this book have designed the explanations to reinforce and supplement the information tested by the questions. If, after reading the explanations for a given chapter, you feel you need still more information about the material covered, you should consult and study the references indicated.

Medicine

PreTest®
Self-Assessment
and Review

Allergy and Immunology

DIRECTIONS: Each question below contains five suggested responses. Select the one **best** response to each question.

1. Which of the following statements about the administration and use of intravenous gamma globulin is correct?

(A) The administration of high doses may produce a remission in idiopathic thrombocytopenic purpura

(B) It must be administered slowly, as concentrated gamma globulin used intravenously has spontaneous anticomplementary activity

(C) Intravenous gamma globulin preparations are safe and effective in the management of patients with selective IgA deficiency

(D) Intravenous gamma globulin preparations have been associated with the development of acquired immune deficiency syndrome (AIDS)

(E) In calculating the dose of intravenous gamma globulin to be administered, the physician should take into account the fact that the half-life of the immunoglobulin in the product is 7 to 12 days in vivo

2. Each of the following statements concerning the stimulation of immunologic responses after vaccine administration is true EXCEPT

(A) a primary immunologic response is first detected within 1 week of the administration of vaccine

(B) repeat exposure to the antigen present in the vaccine causes a secondary immunologic response involving the production of comparable levels of IgM (immunoglobulin M) and IgG

(C) the immunologic response to vaccine administration requires T-cell help to induce B cells to produce IgG

(D) primary exposure to the antigen present in the vaccine causes a weaker immunologic response than does secondary or repeat exposure

(E) antibody response peaks 1 to 2 weeks after the initial administration of vaccine

3.   The presence of bacteria in endocardial vegetations in cases of infective
endocarditis stimulates the immune
system to produce nonspecific antibodies. True statements concerning
this phenomenon include all the following EXCEPT

(A) higher concentrations of circula-
     tory immune complexes correlate
     with extracardiac manifestations
(B) 50 percent of patients develop
     rheumatoid factor
(C) lowest levels of hemolytic com-
     plement are found in cases with
     associated immune complex
     glomerulonephritis
(D) antisarcolemmal antibodies are
     rarely found in patients with sub-
     acute bacterial endocarditis
(E) false positive tests for syphilis
     occasionally occur

4.   Selective IgA deficiency is the
most common of all immunodeficiency
states. Study of patients who have this
problem has revealed that

(A) they may suffer anaphylactic reac-
     tions following the administration
     of serum products
(B) clinical improvement follows regu-
     lar infusions of fresh plasma
(C) secretory component is usually
     increased in an attempt to com-
     pensate for lack of secretory IgA
(D) there is an increase in 19S IgM in
     the secretions of certain affected
     patients
(E) few of them have associated auto-
     immune disorders

5.   True statements concerning the
relationship of asthma and immediate
hypersensitivity (allergic) reactions
include all the following EXCEPT

(A) immediate hypersensitivity reac-
     tions to food allergens are
     involved in provoking asthma in
     an estimated 20 percent of adult
     asthmatics
(B) immediate hypersensitivity reac-
     tions to aeroallergens are involved
     in provoking asthma in an estimated
     25 percent of adult asthmatics
(C) inhalation of a specific allergen in
     a sensitive person can increase
     nonspecific bronchial
     hyperreactivity
(D) after inhalation of allergen, an iso-
     lated, late-phase pulmonary
     response may occur in up to 50
     percent of asthmatics
(E) allergen-provoked asthma is more
     common in children and young
     adults than in older adults

6.   An immunologic basis for atopic
dermatitis is suggested by the fact that
the majority of patients have a family
history of other atopic disorders.
Which of the following statements
concerning this disease is true?

(A) It is ruled out by normal serum
     IgE levels
(B) Patients are susceptible to in-
     fection with herpes simplex and
     Staphylococcus aureus
(C) Cell-mediated immune function is
     usually normal
(D) Total CH_{50} correlates with disease
     activity
(E) There is a higher incidence of con-
     tact dermatitis from poison ivy

7. During the primary immune response a network of interactions is required for the successful elimination of antigen. During this process, which of the following occurs?

(A) CD8-positive T lymphocytes stimulate macrophages to release interleukin 2

(B) CD4-positive T lymphocytes stimulate macrophages to release interleukin 1

(C) B lymphocytes react with antigen and interleukin 1 and then secrete immunoglobulin M (IgM)

(D) Antigen-presenting macrophages present antigen to lymphocyte-activating macrophages

(E) IgA antibodies are secreted by plasma cells that have interacted with secretory piece

8. A 55-year-old farmer develops recurrent cough, dyspnea, fever, and myalgia several hours after entering his barn. All the following statements concerning this patient are true EXCEPT

(A) testing of pulmonary function several hours after an exposure will most likely reveal a restrictive pattern

(B) immediate-type IgE hypersensitivity is not involved in the pathogenesis of his illness

(C) the etiologic agents may well be thermophilic actinomycete antigens

(D) demonstrating precipitable antibodies to the offending antigen confirms the diagnosis of hypersensitivity pneumonitis

(E) a suppressor-cell functional defect is present

9. Which of the following statements concerning allergic reactions in patients receiving penicillin is true?

(A) Allergic reactions occur in approximately 20 percent of patients receiving penicillin

(B) Approximately 25 percent of patients allergic to penicillin will also experience allergic reactions to cephalosporins

(C) Low titers of IgM antibodies specific for the "major" antigenic determinant can be detected in almost every person who has received penicillin

(D) Immediate allergic reactions to penicillin, including anaphylaxis, are most commonly due to the presence of IgE specific for the "major" determinant

(E) The oral route of administration of penicillin is the most likely to induce anaphylaxis

10. All the following statements concerning the immunologic features of active sarcoidosis are true EXCEPT

(A) there are increased levels of helper T lymphocytes at sites of disease activity

(B) patients exhibit cutaneous anergy

(C) there is polyclonal elevation of serum immunoglobulins

(D) peripheral lymphocytosis is characteristic

(E) there is an elevated level of circulating immune complexes

11. A 15-year-old girl presents with a clinical syndrome that is indistinguishable from viral hepatitis; however, her history and serologic findings do not support a viral etiology for her problem. Liver biopsy reveals an established active cirrhosis and hepatocellular necrosis associated with a heavy infiltrate of plasma cells and lymphocytes. Which of the following statements about this girl's condition is most likely to be true?

(A) B lymphocytes are likely to carry the histocompatibility antigen B7
(B) She probably has a polyclonal elevation of IgG
(C) She probably has antimitochondrial antibodies
(D) High titers of anti–smooth muscle antibodies are likely to appear transiently at the onset of her illness
(E) She will probably recover spontaneously after 6 months of illness

12. A 6-year-old white boy presents to his physician with a history of recurrent staphylococcal infections and chronic dermatitis. If the boy has the hyper-IgE syndrome, it is likely that

(A) his IgE level (normally less than 300 ng/mL) will be moderately elevated to between 1000 and 4000 ng/mL
(B) he will have a tendency to develop osteomyelitis
(C) he will have associated asthma or allergic rhinitis
(D) depressed cell-mediated immunity will be discovered
(E) he will respond well to treatment with gamma interferon

13. A 32-year-old woman experiences a severe anaphylactic reaction following a sting from a hornet. Correct statements about this patient include all the following EXCEPT that

(A) she has a strong likelihood of having a similar reaction to a sting from a yellow jacket
(B) she would have a prior history of an adverse reaction to an insect sting
(C) as an adult she is more likely to die as a result of an insect sting than a child with the same history
(D) she should be skin-tested with venom antigens and, if positive, immunotherapy should be started
(E) she most likely began to experience symptoms within 15 min of the sting

DIRECTIONS: Each question below contains four suggested responses of which **one or more** is correct. Select

A	if	**1, 2, and 3**	are correct
B	if	**1 and 3**	are correct
C	if	**2 and 4**	are correct
D	if	**4**	is correct
E	if	**1, 2, 3, and 4**	are correct

14. Correct statements about cryoglobulins include which of the following?

(1) They cannot activate the complement cascade
(2) They are found in most normal people
(3) They are rarely demonstrable in patients with biliary cirrhosis
(4) Clinical symptoms include palpable purpura and peripheral ulcers

15. A 15-year-old boy develops painless hematuria, myalgias, and malaise immediately following a viral upper respiratory infection. Renal biopsy reveals a focal and segmental proliferative glomerulonephritis with mesangial matrix increase and hypercellularity; immunofluorescence reveals diffuse staining for IgA and C3 in all mesangial areas. True statements about this boy's condition include that

(1) depressed levels of C3 and C4 are commonly found
(2) subendothelial and subepithelial deposits are associated with more severe disease
(3) early steroid therapy alters the natural history of the illness
(4) after 25 years, 50 percent of patients will have developed end-stage renal disease

16. True statements regarding immunologic and inflammatory responses to glucocorticoid therapy include which of the following?

(1) There are fewer infectious complications with alternate-day therapy than with daily steroid therapy
(2) Chronic steroid administration causes lymphocytopenia and eosinopenia, but not monocytopenia
(3) High-dose steroid therapy causes a decrease in immunoglobulin levels
(4) Permanent damage to the immunologic system occurs with long term steroid therapy

17. Allergic bronchopulmonary aspergillosis is associated with which of the following statements?

(1) Forty percent of sputum cultures are negative for *Aspergillus fumigatus*
(2) It may lead to pulmonary fibrosis if left untreated
(3) Sputum and blood eosinophilia are characteristic
(4) IgE levels fluctuate with disease activity

18. Disorders associated with circulating blood eosinophilia include

(1) atopic dermatitis
(2) Addison's disease
(3) helminthic infections
(4) protozoan infections

19. Which of the following medications would have an equal effect on both the early (immediate) asthmatic response and the late asthmatic response?

(1) Corticosteroids
(2) Albuterol
(3) Theophylline
(4) Sodium cromolyn

20. Bone marrow–derived B lymphocytes exhibit which of the following characteristics?

(1) They are the proliferating cells in chronic lymphocytic leukemia
(2) They carry a surface membrane receptor for the Fc portion of IgG
(3) They carry a surface membrane receptor for the breakdown products of the third component of complement
(4) They have a receptor for the Epstein-Barr virus

DIRECTIONS: Each group of questions below consists of lettered headings followed by a set of numbered items. For each numbered item select the **one** lettered heading with which it is **most** closely associated. Each lettered heading may be used **once, more than once, or not at all.**

Questions 21–24

For each of the following immunologic diseases, select the immune defect that is most likely to be associated with that disease.

(A) Decreased immunoglobulins
(B) Decreased IgA in secretions
(C) Decreased antibodies to Epstein-Barr virus (EBV) nuclear antigen
(D) Giant cytoplasmic lysosomes in white cells
(E) Abnormal phagocytic respiratory burst

21. Secretory component deficiency

22. Common variable hypogammaglobulinemia

23. Chronic granulomatous disease of childhood

24. X-linked lymphoproliferative disease

Questions 25–28

For each of the following disorders, select the feature with which it is most closely associated.

(A) C1 esterase inhibitor
(B) Peyer's patches
(C) Rheumatoid factor
(D) Allergic reactions to iodides
(E) Sympathetic ophthalmia

25. Rheumatoid arthritis

26. Systemic lupus erythematosus

27. Sjögren's syndrome

28. Leprosy

Questions 29–33

For each of the following diseases, select the HLA antigen that is most closely associated.

    (A) HLA–B27
    (B) HLA–DR4
    (C) HLA–DR3
    (D) HLA–DR2

29. Reiter's syndrome

30. Multiple sclerosis

31. Ankylosing spondylitis

32. Rheumatoid arthritis

33. Systemic lupus erythematosus

Questions 34–38

Match each of the following characteristics with the immunoglobulin type that it best describes.

    (A) IgG
    (B) IgA
    (C) IgM
    (D) IgE
    (E) IgD

34. Binding to high-affinity receptors on mast cells via the Fc receptor

35. The only class of immunoglobulin that crosses the placenta

36. The most efficient complement-fixing immunoglobulin

37. The predominant immunoglobulin in membrane secretions

38. Four subclasses with differences in their heavy chains

DIRECTIONS: The group of questions below consists of four lettered headings followed by a set of numbered items. For each numbered item select

A	if the item is associated with	(A) **only**
B	if the item is associated with	(B) **only**
C	if the item is associated with	**both** (A) and (B)
D	if the item is associated with	**neither** (A) nor (B)

Each lettered heading may be used **once, more than once, or not at all.**

Questions 39–43

    (A) Bullous pemphigoid
    (B) Pemphigus vulgaris
    (C) Both
    (D) Neither

39. Acantholysis

40. Anti–basement membrane zone antibodies

41. Positive Nikolsky's sign

42. Treatment with immunosuppressive drugs

43. Autoimmune disorders

Allergy and Immunology

Answers

1. The answer is A. *(Stiehm, Ann Intern Med 107:367–382, 1987. Wilson, ed 12. p 1402.)* The availability of concentrated forms of gamma globulin suitable for intravenous use represents a significant advance in the management of immuno-deficiency states. Immune serum globulin (ISG) could not be given intravenously, as the aggregates in the material have spontaneous anticomplementary activity and would cause an anaphylactic-like reaction; intravenous preparations of gamma globulin do not have spontaneous anticomplementary activity but do retain the ability to activate the classic complement cascade after combining with antigen. Intravenous gamma globulin can be administered to premature babies who have low immunoglobulin levels because of poor transplacental passage of maternal IgG. Apart from its obvious use in the management of congenital and acquired hypo-gammaglobulinemia, intravenous gamma globulin provides the preferable way of replacing gamma globulin in patients who are severely burned, who have hypo-gammaglobulinemia secondary to chronic lymphocytic leukemia or multiple mye-loma, and who need IgG after plasmapheresis. Patients with selective IgA defi-ciency may make IgE anti-IgA antibodies that could produce an immediate hypersensitivity reaction to intravenous gamma globulin. The product is prepared from pooled plasma obtained at numerous collection sites, thus ensuring that anti-bodies to ubiquitous antigens are represented in each batch of the product. Neither AIDS nor hepatitis has been associated with its use. The half-life of the IgG in the product is approximately 27 days, so it can be administered on a monthly basis. Although the mechanisms are as yet unknown, it is of interest that high doses of intravenous gamma globulin (1 g/kg over 5 days) will produce remission in both acute and chronic idiopathic thrombocytopenic purpura in many patients. In addi-tion, its administration has led to remission in autoimmune neutropenia.

2. The answer is B. *(Bart, J Allergy Clin Immunol 79:296–315, 1987.)* Active immunization involves the administration of an antigen into a host to induce an immunologic response. This antigen may be live organisms, detoxified bacterial toxins, or structural components of the organisms. After the vaccine is administered, there is a several-day latency period before a primary immunologic response is detectable. B cells initially produce IgM and later switch to produce IgG. Although some antigens may be T cell–independent, the switch to IgG synthesis requires T-cell help. Upon reintroduction of the same antigen, a secondary immunologic response occurs. This response, which consists solely of IgG, occurs sooner and is more intense than the primary response. Measuring the level of circulating anti bodies present after vaccination gives an indication of the adequacy of the immunologic response. However, the presence of antibodies does not always insure clinical protection.

3.   The answer is D.   *(Hurst, ed 7. pp 1238–1239.)* While the symptoms of subacute endocarditis develop insidiously, the clinical and laboratory manifestations may be grouped under three categories: as evidence of a systemic infection, an intravascular lesion, or an immunologic reaction to infection. As noted, the presence of bacteria in endocardial vegetations stimulates the production of nonspecific antibodies leading to polyclonal increases in gamma globulins, positive rheumatoid factor, occasional false positive tests for syphilis, and decreased complement. Circulating immune complexes have been detected in the vast majority of patients; higher concentrations correlate with the presence of arthritis, splenomegaly, and glomerulonephritis. Antiendocardial and antisarcolemmal antibodies are found in 60 to 100 percent of cases. By history, manifestations of immunologic reactions include arthralgia, myalgia, and tenosynovitis; physical examination reveals arthritis, signs of uremia, vascular phenomena, and finger clubbing.

4.   The answer is A.   *(Wilson, ed 12. p 1400.)* IgA deficiency occurs in approximately 1 out of 700 births. Failure to produce this antibody results in recurrent upper respiratory tract infections in 50 percent of affected patients. IgA-deficient patients frequently have autoimmune disorders, atopic problems, and malabsorption and eventually develop pulmonary disease. Replacement therapy is entirely unsatisfactory. If IgA is totally absent, its administration can represent an antigenic challenge that may result in anaphylaxis. Secretory component is normally present, and very few cases of IgA deficiency are due to a lack of this accessory factor. Some patients compensate for IgA deficiency by secreting a low-molecular-weight 7S IgM antibody.

5.   The answer is A.   *(Middleton, ed 3. pp 230–236, 1063–1092.)* Asthma is a reversible obstructive airway disease characterized by edema, hypersecretion, and hyperresponsive airways. It can be categorized as intrinsic or extrinsic. Intrinsic asthma is due to nonspecific physical triggers and respiratory infections. In extrinsic asthma, exposure to inhalant allergens and, rarely, to foods triggers an immediate hypersensitivity reaction. Both types of asthma may be present in the same patient. In extrinsic asthma, allergen triggers either immediate or late-phase responses or, more commonly, both. The immediate response involves IgE on mast cells reacting with allergen and causing mediator release. This reaction begins 10 to 20 min after exposure to allergen and resolves within 1 to 2 h. IgE may also be involved in the late-phase response and cause mediator release, which attracts inflammatory cells to the area. A late-phase response begins 3 to 4 h after exposure and persists for up to 12 h or longer.

12   Medicine

6.   The answer is B. *(Fitzpatrick, ed 3. pp 1385-1408. Hanifin, J Allergy Clin Immunol 73:211-222, 1984.)* Atopic dermatitis is a chronic relapsing inflammation of the skin characterized by pruritus accompanied by papules, lichenification, and eczematous lesions. The lesions are located mainly on the head and neck of infants and on the flexural areas of older children and adults. There are no diagnostic histologic or laboratory features; therefore, the diagnosis is based upon clinical features. There is typically a personal or family history of asthma, hay fever, or eczema and onset is usually in the childhood years. All patients have xerosis and are susceptible to pyogenic infections, especially those caused by *Staphylococcus aureus*, viral infections primarily due to herpes simplex and vaccinia, and superficial fungal infections. While IgE levels may be normal, they are typically elevated in patients with severe atopic dermatitis. Additionally, a defect in cell-mediated immunity exists and manifests as an increased susceptibility to cutaneous infections, a lower incidence of contact dermatitis from poison ivy, and a reduced rate of sensitization to dinitrochlorobenzene. The natural history of the disease is variable; 10 percent of patients overall will have persistent dermatitis that remains unchanged or worsens while the vast majority will improve. Treatment involves antihistamines for pruritus, antibiotics for secondary infections, and topical steroids.

7.   The answer is B. *(Roitt, ed 2. pp 8.1-8.12. Wilson, ed 12. pp 76-86.)* The primary immune response involves an initial presentation of antigen to a CD4 inducer T cell by an antigen-presenting macrophage. The latter cell is remarkable for the strong expression of HLA–D histocompatibility molecules on its membrane. T cells, in contrast to B cells, are able to recognize antigen only in the presence of HLA molecules. The macrophage is thus able to present both foreignness (antigen) and self (HLA–D) to a CD4 inducer T cell, an essential step in initiating the immune response. T lymphocytes carrying the surface antigen CD4 (detected by monoclonal antibodies) bind to the HLA–D/antigen complex and then activate the macrophages known as lymphocyte-activating macrophages. These cells release interleukin 1, a messenger substance that binds to a receptor on the surface of the CD4-positive T cell. The CD4-positive T cell then releases interleukin 2, a second soluble messenger substance that causes the activated T cell to proliferate and produce other classes of interleukins that act on activated B cells to stimulate antibody production. Interleukin 2 also binds directly to B cells that have recognized antigen and induces them to mature into plasma cells that will secrete antibody.

8.   The answer is D. *(Levy, Ann Allergy 54:167-171, 1985.)* Hypersensitivity pneumonitis is characterized by an immunologic inflammatory reaction in response to inhaling organic dusts, the most common of which are thermophilic actinomycetes, fungi, and avian proteins. In the acute form of the illness, exposure to the offending antigen is intense. Cough, dyspnea, fever, chills, and myalgia, which typically occur 4 to 8 h after exposure, are the presenting symptoms. In the subacute form, antigen exposure is moderate, chills and fever are usually absent, and cough, anorexia, weight loss, and dyspnea dominate the presentation. In the chronic form of hypersensitivity pneumonitis, progressive dyspnea, weight loss, and anorexia are seen; pulmonary fibrosis is a noted complication. In most cases, leukocytosis and eosinophilia are present; the finding of IgG antibody to the offending antigen is universal although it may be present in asymptomatic patients as well and is therefore not diagnostic. While peripheral T-cell, B-cell, and monocyte counts are normal, a suppressor-cell functional defect can be demonstrated in these patients. Inhalation challenge with the suspected antigen and concomitant testing of pulmonary function help to confirm the diagnosis. Therapy involves avoidance; steroids are administered in severe cases. Bronchodilators and antihistamines are not effective.

9.   The answer is C. *(Patterson, ed 3. pp 595–606.)* One to three percent of patients being treated with penicillin will experience an allergic reaction to the drug. The reaction usually occurs in the first 3 weeks of treatment and is most common when therapy is resumed after an interruption. Allergic reactions can occur with any route of administration; however, anaphylactic or severe generalized allergic reactions are more common when penicillin is given parenterally. Penicillin reactions are of three types: (1) immediate reactions begin within 1 h of administering the drug and usually involve urticaria or anaphylaxis; (2) accelerated reactions begin 1 to 72 h after the drug is given and are manifest as urticaria or angioedema; and (3) delayed or late reactions begin more than 72 h after drug administration and typically involve skin eruptions. It is the degradation products of penicillin that bind to serum proteins to form immunogens. Ninety-five percent of penicillin binds with protein to form the benzylpenicilloyl (BPO) group, or "major" determinant. The majority of antibodies formed in penicillin-allergic persons are specific for this determinant. About 5 percent of penicillin is degraded to various "minor" determinants, which include penicilloates and benzylpenicillin itself. In general, immediate reactions, including anaphylaxis, are usually due to IgE antibodies specific for the "minor" determinants. In contrast, accelerated and late reactions are usually secondary to IgE specific to the "major" determinants. Accelerated reactions involve preformed IgE, while in late reactions, IgE is formed during the course of the treatment. One-third of patients with late-reaction skin eruptions have been found to have IgM specific for the "major" determinant. Skin testing to diagnose penicillin allergy is done to both the "major" and "minor" determinants. The "major" determinant is commercially available as benzylpenicilloyl-polylysine (Pre-Pen). The "minor" determinants are tested with either benzylpenicillin G or a "minor" determinant mixture. The mixture is not commercially available. In patients with a positive history of penicillin allergy, approximately 7 to 10 percent will experience an allergic reaction to cephalosporins.

10.   The answer is D. *(Fink, JAMA 258:2943–2944, 1987.)* Sarcoidosis is a multisystem granulomatous disorder characterized by bilateral hilar lymphadenopathy; pulmonary infiltrates; skin lesions; peripheral lymphadenopathy; ocular disease including iridocyclitis, keratoconjunctivitis, and chorioretinitis; hepatosplenomegaly; and neurologic, cardiac, and musculoskeletal involvement. Studies of patients with active sarcoidosis reveal immunologic abnormalities, features of which are cutaneous anergy and a hyperactive humoral system. A polyclonal elevation of immunoglobulins is found and depressed numbers of circulating T lymphocytes are characteristic. Sarcoidosis is characterized by spontaneous remissions; active disease usually responds to steroid therapy.

11.   The answer is B. *(Strober, JAMA 258:2962-2969, 1987.)* The patient presented in the question probably has autoimmune chronic active hepatitis, a disease of unknown etiology characterized by the chronic presence of circulating autoantibodies, such as anti-smooth muscle antibody, and severe hypergammaglobulinemia with polyclonal increase in IgG. Antimitochondrial antibodies exist in 10 to 30 percent of affected patients. This is in contrast to primary biliary cirrhosis, which has elevated serum IgM and, in 90 percent of patients, increased antimitochondrial antibody titers. Chronic active hepatitis is infrequently associated with thyroid and gastric autoimmune disorders. There is an increased incidence of HLA-B8 in patients with this disease. The disease has a variable course with some patients having long remissions. Corticosteroids have been shown to prolong survival.

12.   The answer is D. *(Middleton, ed 3. pp 300-301.)* The hyper-IgE syndrome (formerly known as Job's syndrome) affects both males and females by causing chronic dermatitis and increased susceptibility to infections with staphylococcal organisms. Sensitivity to candidal and streptococcal infections can also occur. The recurrent infections are found to mainly affect the skin and respiratory tract, leading to the formation of abscesses and pneumatoceles. The condition is associated with extremely high serum IgE levels, often greater than 10,000 ng/mL. Blood and sputum eosinophilia also occurs. Most polymorphonuclear cell functions are normal, with defects in chemotaxis discovered in some patients. Most patients have deficient cell-mediated immune function. An autosomal dominant form of inheritance appears to be involved in this syndrome. Treatment consists of penicillinase-resistant penicillin and surgical drainage of abscesses.

13.   The answer is B. *(Middleton, ed 3. pp 1345-1352.)* The incidence of insect sting allergy is difficult to determine. Approximately 40 deaths per year occur as a result of Hymenoptera stings. Additional fatalities undoubtedly occur and are unknowingly attributed to other causes. Both atopic and nonatopic persons experience reactions to insect stings. The responses range from large local reactions with erythema and swelling at the sting site to acute anaphylaxis. The majority of fatal reactions occur in adults, with most persons having had no previous reaction to a stinging insect. Reactions can occur with the first sting and usually begin within 15 min. Enzymes, biogenic amines, and peptides are the allergens present in the insects' venom that provoke allergic reactions. Venoms are commercially available for testing and treatment. Within the Vespidae family—consisting of hornets, yellow jackets, and wasps—cross-sensitivity to the various insect venoms occurs. The honeybee, which belongs to the Apid family, does not show cross-reactivity with the vespids. Patients with systemic reactions are skin-tested with venom concentrations of up to 1 μg/mL. Greater concentrations tend to cause nonspecific skin reactions. Venom immunotherapy is indicated for patients with a history of sting anaphylaxis and positive skin tests.

14.   The answer is C (2, 4). *(Grieco, pp 92–99.)* Cryoglobulins are immuno-globulins that exhibit reversible precipitation in the cold. They may be *simple*, in which case they are of one immunoglobulin class, monoclonal, and almost always associated with multiple myeloma or macroglobulinemia; or *mixed*, in which case they are of more than one immunoglobulin class, either monoclonal or polyclonal, and usually found to be rheumatoid factor. While cryoglobulins occur in most normal people, they do so in low levels and are always polyclonal; pathologic cryoglobulins occur at concentrations of greater than 0.2 mg/mL. Associations include vasculitis, glomerulonephritis, collagen diseases, subacute bacterial endo-carditis, syphilis, chronic HBV infection, and infectious mononucleosis. The finding of a monoclonal immunoglobulin should raise the possibility of an underlying lymphoproliferative or plasma cell disorder; IgM monoclonals are particularly asso-ciated with chronic lymphocytic leukemia (CLL), lymphoma, and angioblastic lymphadenopathy. Treatment is directed toward the underlying illness although plasmapheresis may be effective in the short term. Idiopathic mixed cryo-globulinemia may respond to cytotoxic drugs with amelioration of the associated nephritis, arthritis, and purpura.

15.   The answer is C (2, 4). *(Wilson, ed 12. p 1179.)* Berger's disease (IgA nephropathy), the most common cause of recurrent hematuria of glomerular origin, usually affects young adult males. It is typically preceded by a viral illness. The hematuria may be gross or microscopic and the proteinuria is usually less than 3.5 g per day although the nephrotic syndrome is occasionally seen. Diagnosis is based on finding diffuse mesangial deposition of IgA usually accompanied by C3 and less frequently by IgG; C1q and C4 are not found. Fifty percent of patients have elevated levels of IgA, while serum complement levels remain normal. A poor prognosis is associated with azotemia, hypertension, and the nephrotic syndrome at the time of diagnosis and subepithelial and subendothelial deposits on renal biopsy. The disease generally progresses slowly and no form of therapy has been shown to be effective.

16.   The answer is B (1, 3). *(Felig, ed 2. pp 548–551, 795.)* In general terms, glucocorticoids affect cellular processes, leukocyte distribution, and macrophages more than they affect humoral processes, leukocyte function, and polymorphonuclear leukocytes. Circulating lymphocytes, monocytes, and eosinophils are decreased secondary to redistribution of these cells into other compartments, while blood polymorphonuclear cells are increased. Within 2 h of administration of steroids, there is a decrease in inflammatory cell accumulation at sites of injury. Lymphocyte proliferation, mediator production, autologous and allogenic mixed leukocyte reactions, and cutaneous delayed hypersensitivity are all suppressed. While there is no evidence that complement components are lowered, a small decrease in immunoglobulins secondary to decreased synthesis and increased catabolism is observed. Because precursor cells are steroid resistant, permanent damage to the immunologic system does not occur. The cushingoid effects of glucocorticoid therapy can be minimized by administering the full 48-h dose as a *single* dose of intermediate-acting steroid on the morning of every other day. However, this transition from daily to alternate-day administration should be attempted only after the manifestations of the disease are reasonably under control and is best made gradually.

17.   The answer is E (all). *(Greenberger, Ann Allergy 56:444-448, 1986.)* Aspergillus is a ubiquitous fungus that is usually acquired by inhalation of its spores. While exposure is almost universal, disease is uncommon. Allergic bronchopulmonary aspergillosis is usually a complication of preexisting asthma and is characterized by transient pulmonary infiltrates, sputum and blood eosinophilia, elevated serum IgE, and an immediate-type skin-test response to *Aspergillus* antigen. Patients present complaining of fevers, chills, malaise, and a productive cough. If left untreated, bronchiectasis and pulmonary fibrosis are possible complications. Corticosteroids are the mainstay of therapy. Because evidence indicates that elevations in IgE occur prior to clinical exacerbations, prevention of acute flares is possible with early use of steroids.

18.   The answer is A (1, 2, 3). *(Middleton, ed 3. pp 861-890.)* Increased numbers of eosinophils in circulating blood are associated with various inflammatory, neoplastic, infectious, and allergic diseases. Normal, healthy adults have a blood eosinophilia of approximately 100 to 125 cells per cubic millimeter. Obvious conditions that are associated with increased blood eosinophilia include hypereosinophilic syndrome and eosinophilic gastroenteritis. Eosinophilia may be a manifestation of an adverse reaction to drugs such as penicillin, phenytoin, sulfonamides, and L-tryptophan. Parasitic infections due to helminths provoke eosinophilic reactions, while protozoan infections do not. The parasites must have a tissue invasive phase in their life cycles in order to provoke this reaction. Eosinophilia frequently accompanies atopic disorders such as asthma and atopic dermatitis. In addition, peripheral eosinophilia is seen with endocrine disorders, such as Addison's disease, and with various connective tissue diseases involving fascia, muscle, or synovium.

19.   The answer is D (4). *(O'Byrne, Am Rev Respir Dis 136:740-751, 1987.)* Inhalation of an allergen by a sensitized person leads to a distinct series of events.

Within 10 min of the exposure, bronchoconstriction occurs, which continues for 1 to 3 h. This is termed the early, or immediate, asthmatic response. In most asthmatics, this is followed 3 to 4 h after exposure by the late asthmatic response, which may last for 24 h or more. The immediate response occurs secondary to the interaction of allergen with mast cell–bound IgE, causing mediator release. The late asthmatic response is also believed to be IgE-dependent. However, in addition to the effects of mast cell or basophil mediators, the late response involves airway inflammation with eosinophils and neutrophils predominating. The difference in mechanisms of the early and late responses accounts for their different reactions to various medications. Albuterol and other β-receptor agonists inhibit the early asthmatic response, but have little or no effect on the late response. Theophylline slightly decreases the immediate response and has a significant effect on the late response. Corticosteroids have a minimal effect on the immediate response, while inhibiting the late response. In contrast, sodium cromolyn inhibits both the early and late responses.

20.   The answer is E (all). *(Roitt, ed 2. pp 2.6–2.7. Wilson, ed 12. p 79.)* B lymphocytes are cells that mature in the bone marrow and have surface receptors that bind the Fc portion of IgG, some complement components, the Epstein-Barr virus, and, most importantly, specific antigen. The last is accomplished via a specific immunoglobulin receptor molecule. The cells have a short half-life (days) and are thus quite different from T cells that live for years. Oncogenic influence may cause these cells to proliferate and produce chronic lymphocytic leukemia or lymphomas. B cells bind antigen and then divide to form plasma cells. The cells secrete an antibody product identical to that of the receptor on the B cell from which it was derived.

21–24.   The answers are: 21-B, 22-A, 23-E, 24-C. *(Buckley, JAMA 258:2841–2850, 1987.)* IgA is present in serum as a monomer and in secretions as a polymer consisting of two basic IgA units, a J chain and a secretory component. The secretory component is synthesized by epithelial cells near mucous membranes and may function to transport IgA across the mucosa and into secretions. Patients with secretory component deficiency will have a normal serum IgA level with a lack of IgA in secretions. These patients develop chronic intestinal candidiasis and diarrhea.

Patients with common variable hypogammaglobulinemia are usually well until 15 to 35 years of age. They then develop pyogenic infections and have increased incidence of autoimmune diseases. Other associated conditions include a spruelike syndrome, giardiasis, gastric atrophy, bronchiectasis, and pernicious anemia. Most patients with this disease have a defect in B-cell differentiation. Normal numbers of circulating immunoglobulin-bearing B cells are present but they do not differentiate into immunoglobulin-producing plasma cells. About 10 percent of patients with this condition have associated T-cell abnormalities.

Chronic granulomatous disease of childhood is an X-linked disorder with onset of symptoms during the first 2 years of life. Neutrophils and monocytes from these patients have a normal ability to phagocytize organisms but have abnormal O_2-

dependent killing of catalase-positive organisms (e.g., *Staphylococcus aureus*, *Proteus*) owing to a defect in the intracellular respiratory burst enzyme complex. Defects in both cytochrome b-245 and NADPH oxidase have been identified. Patients develop pneumonia, skin infections, draining adenopathy, osteomyelitis, and abscesses.

X-linked lymphoproliferative disease or Duncan's syndrome is characterized by a poor immune response to infection with Epstein-Barr virus (EBV). Patients with this disease are well until they develop infectious mononucleosis; two-thirds have a fatal outcome. Of those surviving the acute infection, a majority will develop hypogammaglobulinemia, B-cell lymphomas, or both. Patients have an impaired antibody response to EBV nuclear antigen. Other nonspecific immune defects, such as decreased natural killer cell function, increased percentage of CD8-positive T cells, and abnormal lymphocyte proliferation in response to mitogens, occur.

25-28. The answers are: 25-C, 26-C, 27-C, 28-C. *(Wilson, ed 12. p 1439.)* Rheumatoid factor usually is an IgM antibody that has activity against aggregated or altered IgG, although rheumatoid factors of all immunoglobulin classes have been described. Rheumatoid factors are autoantibodies, and it seems certain that the macromolecular immune complexes so formed can activate complement mechanisms and cause joint damage. The activation of the complement cascade results in polymorphonuclear leukocyte infiltration into the joint fluid with subsequent damage to synovial tissues.

Though most frequently found in adult rheumatoid arthritis (90 percent), rheumatoid factors are also found in juvenile rheumatoid arthritis (25 percent), Sjögren's syndrome (75 percent), systemic lupus erythematosus (30 percent), and occasionally other inflammatory diseases, including leprosy and infectious mononucleosis. It is possible that an infectious agent generates an aggregated or altered antibody to that agent, and that this changed immunoglobulin stimulates the production of rheumatoid factor in the susceptible person.

Rheumatoid arthritis can occur in agammaglobulinemic persons who by definition are incapable of making rheumatoid factors; it can also occur in a seronegative form in which no autoantibodies can be found. Usually such cases are milder than the seropositive cases of rheumatoid arthritis, but they raise the possibility that mechanisms other than the activation of complement by rheumatoid complexes may be important in the immunopathogenesis of rheumatoid arthritis.

29-33. The answers are: 29-A, 30-D, 31-A, 32-B, 33-C. *(Wilson, ed 12. pp 86-92.)* The major histocompatibility complex is contained on the short arm of chromosome 6 and codes for three classes of cell-surface antigens. Class I antigens, consisting of HLA-A, -B and -C, are found on virtually all nucleated cells. Class II antigens, referred to as HLA-D/DR, are expressed on B lymphocytes, activated T lymphocytes, and monocytes. Another group of antigens, belonging to class III, consists of the C2, C4, and factor B components of complement. HLA antigens play a role in immune recognition. For example, T lymphocytes recognize antigen in conjunction with HLA antigens. There is an increased risk of susceptibility to certain diseases in people possessing particular HLA antigens. For example, HLA-B27 is found in only 7 percent of people of Western European ancestry, yet is present in 80 to 90 percent of patients with ankylosing spondylitis.

34-38. The answers are: 34-D, 35-A, 36-C, 37-B, 38-A. *(Stites, ed 6. pp 27-34.)* Mature plasma cells produce immunoglobulins capable of combining with antigenic determinants on diverse substances. Immunoglobulins constitute approximately 20 percent of all plasma proteins. They have a basic structure composed of four polypeptide chains—two light and two heavy chains. Light chains are of two types—kappa and lambda. There are five classes of heavy chains—gamma, alpha, mu, delta, and epsilon. The type of heavy chains an immunoglobulin possesses determines its class. The various classes of immunoglobulins are present in serum in different amounts and have different properties.

IgG constitutes 70 percent of the total serum immunoglobulins and is present as four subclasses. IgG is capable of crossing the placenta and fixing serum complement. It is the major immunoglobulin involved in secondary immune responses. IgA represents 15 percent of the total serum immunoglobulins and is the predominant immunoglobulin in membrane secretions. It provides primary immune protection at the mucosal level. IgM exists as a pentameric structure and accounts for 10 percent of normal immunoglobulins. It plays a major role in early immune responses and efficiently activates the classic complement pathway. IgE is present in only trace amounts in serum, but is bound avidly to Fc receptors on mast cells and basophils. When cell-surface IgE is cross-linked by antigen, mediator release occurs and an immediate hypersensitivity reaction ensues. IgD represents less than 1 percent of normal serum immunoglobulins. Many circulating B lymphocytes have IgD on their surfaces, where its function is unclear.

39-43. The answers are: 39-B, 40-A, 41-B, 42-C, 43-C. *(Patel, Ann Allergy 50:144-149, 1984.)* Bullous pemphigoid is characterized by large, tense bullae that have a predilection for the inner thighs, flexor surfaces of the forearms, axillae, groin, and lower abdomen; mucous membranes may be involved, as well. Direct immunofluorescence reveals the presence of autoantibodies against the perilesional skin basement membrane zone in the lamina lucida where cleavage takes place. A mild vasculitis in lesional skin is also noted. While the disease is generally benign and self-limited, therapy with steroids, sometimes in combination with immunosuppressive drugs, is often used to control eruptions; relapses are infrequent. Healing generally takes place without scarring.

Pemphigus refers to a group of bullous diseases that includes pemphigus vulgaris, pemphigus vegitans, pemphigus foliaceus, and fogo selvagem. Pemphigus vulgaris is the most common type seen in North America and is characterized by acantholysis and the presence of IgG directed against cell surface antigenic determinants on keratinocytes. The bullae tend to spread on pressure (positive Nikolsky's sign) to involve large areas and heal poorly. Therapy involves corticosteroids along with steroid-sparing cytotoxic drugs. Recurrences are not infrequent and patients should be followed every 4 to 6 months after cessation of therapy for clinical or serologic recurrence of pemphigus.

Infectious Disease

DIRECTIONS: Each question below contains five suggested responses. Select the **one best** response to each question.

44. All the following statements concerning Rocky Mountain spotted fever are true EXCEPT

(A) fulminant cases leading to death in 5 days have been described
(B) the causative organism creates a vasculitis of small arteries and veins
(C) patients may present with severe abdominal pain
(D) the disease usually begins with a rash
(E) patients recovering from the disease are resistant to reinfection

45. Medical personnel who have just completed mouth-to-mouth resuscitation on a patient with known meningococcemia should receive chemoprophylaxis with which of the following antibiotics?

(A) Penicillin
(B) Rifampin
(C) Sulfadiazine
(D) Erythromycin
(E) None of the above

46. Toxic shock syndrome is characteristically associated with each of the following EXCEPT

(A) fever
(B) hypotension
(C) rash
(D) hypercalcemia
(E) *Staphylococcus aureus*

47. All the following statements concerning cryptococcal meningoencephalitis are true EXCEPT

(A) it may be a presenting manifestation of AIDS
(B) it may occur in patients with no identifiable immunologic defect
(C) urine or blood culture may be positive for the organism
(D) the India ink preparation usually reveals gram-negative bacteria
(E) detection of cryptococcal polysaccharide antigen in cerebrospinal fluid (CSF) is useful in making the diagnosis

48. Patients with cellular immune dysfunction are particularly susceptible to infection with all the following organisms EXCEPT

(A) cytomegalovirus
(B) *Haemophilus influenzae*
(C) *Mycobacterium tuberculosis*
(D) *Pneumocystis carinii*
(E) *Histoplasma capsulatum*

49. A fresh-water swimmer develops macules on his lower extremities 10 h after bathing in an area known to harbor nonhuman cercariae schistosomes. The natural history of the "swimmer's itch" includes

(A) the development of microscopic hematuria in about 2 months
(B) the development of a self-limited dermatitis
(C) the late development of cirrhosis and splenomegaly
(D) rapid abatement of fever after treatment with topical thiabendazole
(E) human-to-human transmission to persons in close physical contact

50. Chagas' disease exhibits all the following findings EXCEPT

(A) esophageal dilatation
(B) megacolon
(C) pancreatic pseudocysts
(D) unilateral conjunctivitis with edema of eyelids and face
(E) subacute myocarditis

51. All the following statements concerning maculopapular rashes associated with infectious diseases are true EXCEPT

(A) *Mycoplasma* infections cause a maculopapular rash characterized by a prominent palmar or plantar involvement
(B) erythema infectiosum is associated with a confluent erythema over the cheeks and symmetric eruptions on the trunk, arms, and legs but rarely on the palms and soles
(C) echoviruses cause a maculopapular rash that may be associated with petechiae
(D) exanthem subitum (roseola infantum) produces a mild maculopapular rash that is largely asymptomatic even though it lasts 5 to 10 days
(E) transient maculopapular rashes occur in typhoid fever

52. Infection by *Plasmodium falciparum* is associated with all the following clinical signs or syndromes EXCEPT

(A) blackwater fever (hemoglobinuric fever)
(B) resistance to 4-aminoquinoline drugs such as chloroquine
(C) febrile episodes occurring every 72 h
(D) cerebral malaria with coma
(E) high-density parasitemia

53. Two days before the end of a 2-week vacation in the Caribbean, a 43-year-old man who had enjoyed good health experiences nausea, flatulence, epigastric discomfort, and watery diarrhea. Three weeks later, the diarrhea having persisted unabated, he consults his physician; the only abnormality found on stool examination is the presence of the trophozoite stages of *Giardia lamblia*. All the following statements concerning the patient's disorder are true EXCEPT that

(A) radiography may reveal irritability of the duodenal bulb
(B) the stools of a homosexual patient's sexual partner may be positive for the same protozoan
(C) the significance of the stool finding is not clear
(D) IgA deficiency, although commonly associated with *Giardia lamblia* infestation, is not likely to be a factor in this case
(E) rapid weight loss associated with the diarrhea would be consistent with a diagnosis of giardiasis

54. In a patient who has mitral valve insufficiency, prophylactic antibiotic treatment is recommended for all the following procedures EXCEPT

(A) cardiac catheterization
(B) prostatectomy
(C) cystoscopy
(D) sigmoidoscopy
(E) endoscopy

55. Rabies, an acute viral disease of the mammalian central nervous system, is transmitted by infective secretions, usually saliva. Which of the following statements about this disease is the most accurate?

(A) The disease is caused by a reovirus that elicits both complement-fixing and hemagglutinating antibodies useful in the diagnosis of the disease
(B) The incubation period is variable and, although 10 days is the most common elapsed time between infection and symptoms, some cases remain asymptomatic for 30 days
(C) Only 30 percent of infected patients will survive
(D) In the United States, the skunk and the raccoon have been important recent sources of human disease
(E) Wild animals that have bitten and are suspected of being rabid should be killed and their brains examined for virus particles by electron microscopy

56. All the following statements concerning herpes simplex encephalitis are true EXCEPT that

(A) it is a common form of nonepidemic adult encephalitis in the United States
(B) the causative virus can usually be isolated from cerebrospinal fluid
(C) the cerebrospinal fluid in affected patients often contains red blood cells during acute illness
(D) it may result in necrosis of brain tissue and high fatality
(E) evidence of a localized brain lesion may be found on electroencephalography

DIRECTIONS: Each question below contains four suggested responses of which **one or more** is correct. Select

A	if	**1, 2, and 3**	are	correct
B	if	**1 and 3**	are	correct
C	if	**2 and 4**	are	correct
D	if	**4**	is	correct
E	if	**1, 2, 3, and 4**	are	correct

57. A lifelong resident of Connecticut traveled to Arizona to work on a water project in the desert. Shortly after beginning work he developed fever, cough, and shortness of breath. He was diagnosed as having *Coccidioides immitis* by urine wet smear and culture. Other findings that he might be expected to develop include

(1) erythema nodosum
(2) arthralgias
(3) pneumonia
(4) erythema multiforme

58. Resistance to antiviral drugs has been demonstrated in the clinical setting of

(1) herpes simplex
(2) cytomegalovirus (CMV)
(3) influenza A
(4) human immunodeficiency virus (HIV)

59. Immunizations that would be recommended for a healthy adult over age 65 who has not been immunized for at least the past 15 years include

(1) pneumococcal vaccine
(2) influenza vaccine
(3) tetanus and diphtheria toxoids (Td)
(4) oral polio vaccine (OPV)

60. Correct statements regarding herpes zoster (shingles) include which of the following?

(1) It probably results from reactivation of latent infection in persons who previously have had chickenpox
(2) It usually causes a bilateral skin eruption in a dermatomal distribution
(3) It is often associated with depression of delayed hypersensitivity by immunosuppressive chemotherapy
(4) Severe pain in an affected dermatome usually precedes the onset of the vesicular lesions and lasts until the skin manifestations clear

61. A patient with end-stage renal disease is maintained on chronic hemodialysis via a prosthetic subcutaneous arteriovenous fistula. Correct statements concerning infections of the conduit include that

(1) most are commonly caused by endogenous *Staphylococcus aureus*
(2) empiric antibiotic therapy should include coverage for *Pseudomonas aeruginosa*
(3) local findings of infection are absent in up to one-third of patients
(4) antibiotic therapy is curative in the vast majority of cases

62. A previously healthy 25-year-old medical student consults you prior to leaving for work in a hospital in tropical Africa. Appropriate topics for discussion include

(1) chemoprophylaxis of malaria
(2) foods and beverages to avoid
(3) measures to reduce exposure to insects
(4) immunization against hepatitis B

63. Infection with influenza A virus may be

(1) treated with an antiviral drug such as amantadine
(2) prevented by an antiviral drug such as amantadine
(3) prevented by immunization
(4) acquired by immunization

64. A diabetic patient who requires insulin is seen in the emergency room with a painfully swollen eye, proptosis, and loss of external eye movements. She is acidotic. Tenderness is elicited over the frontal sinus of the affected side. Rapid involvement of the other eye would suggest which of the following disorders?

(1) Osteomyelitis
(2) Orbital cellulitis
(3) Mucormycosis
(4) Cavernous sinus thrombosis

65. *Streptococcus pneumoniae* is responsible for a significant number of deaths. A vaccine containing capsular polysaccharides from the 23 pneumococcal types responsible for 90 percent of bacteremic pneumococcal infections in the United States is available. Patients who should receive this vaccine include

(1) children who experience, in the first year of life, three attacks of otitis media caused by the pneumococcus
(2) patients with functional or anatomic asplenia
(3) patients with sickle cell disease who have not received a booster dose of vaccine for 2 years
(4) patients over 55 years of age who have chronic cardiovascular disease

66. A 28-year-old woman is brought to an emergency room with an infection in a foot wound sustained 7 days earlier. Examination reveals a moderate degree of cellulitis associated with the wound. Primary immunization at 4 years of age had consisted of three doses of tetanus toxoid and one booster 8 years later. She should now be treated with

(1) wound debridement
(2) diphtheria-pertussis-tetanus vaccine (DPT)
(3) tetanus-diphtheria toxoids (Td)
(4) hyperimmune antitetanus gamma globulin

67. A 36-year-old woman has recently returned to the U.S. after a vacation in Egypt that included several swims in the Nile River. She has developed dysuria and hematuria; eggs of *Schistosoma haematobium* are found in her urine. Correct statements concerning this patient include that

(1) sexual partners are at risk of acquiring infection
(2) praziquantel is the drug of choice
(3) she should use separate toilet facilities until the infection has cleared
(4) if she is not treated, hydronephrosis may occur

68. A 60-year-old man is diagnosed as having *Streptococcus bovis* endocarditis. Appropriate evaluation and treatment should include

(1) throat culture
(2) intravenous penicillin
(3) evaluation for development of rheumatic fever
(4) colonoscopy

69. *Histoplasma capsulatum* is associated with which of the following conditions?

(1) Pneumonia
(2) Pulmonary cavities
(3) Meningitis
(4) Febrile hepatosplenomegaly

70. Antibiotics contraindicated during pregnancy include

(1) trimethoprim-sulfamethoxazole
(2) chloramphenicol
(3) erythromycin estolate
(4) tetracycline

71. Antibiotics associated with pseudo-membranous colitis include

(1) gentamicin
(2) ampicillin
(3) tetracycline
(4) clindamycin

DIRECTIONS: Each group of questions below consists of lettered headings followed by a set of numbered items. For each numbered item select the **one** lettered heading with which it is **most** closely associated. Each lettered heading may be used **once, more than once, or not at all.**

Questions 72–76

For each description of food poisoning that follows, select the microorganism with which it is most closely associated.

    (A) *Clostridium perfringens*
    (B) *Staphylococcus aureus*
    (C) *Shigella sonnei*
    (D) *Vibrio parahaemolyticus*
    (E) *Yersinia enterocolitica*

72. Severe cramps, diarrhea, and occasional nausea and vomiting. Associated with cold or reheated cooked meats, gravy, or stews

73. Severe cramps, bloody diarrhea, and fever. Epidemics associated with contaminated water and food have been reported

74. Moderate to severe cramps, bloody diarrhea, and fever. Epidemics in the United States have been associated with ingestion of contaminated crabs

75. Severe nausea and vomiting within 1 to 6 h of eating. Associated with contaminated meats and dairy products

76. Severe abdominal pain and tenderness that may mimic appendicitis. Outbreaks have been associated with contaminated water

Questions 77–81

Match the following.

    (A) Koplik's spots
    (B) Agammaglobulinemia
    (C) A vesicular and pustular eruption that begins when the patient is afebrile
    (D) Acute cerebellar ataxia
    (E) Pancreatitis

77. Mumps

78. Chickenpox

79. Smallpox

80. Echovirus

81. Measles

Questions 82–86

Match the clinical illness with the appropriate opportunistic pathogen in patients with AIDS.

(A) *Pneumocystis carinii*
(B) *Toxoplasma gondii*
(C) *Cryptosporidium*
(D) Cytomegalovirus
(E) *Salmonella*

82. Pneumonia

83. Retinitis

84. Seizures

85. Bacteremia

86. Diarrhea diagnosed by direct stool examination

Questions 87–90

Match the following.

(A) *Plasmodium vivax*
(B) *Plasmodium malariae*
(C) *Plasmodium falciparum*
(D) *Plasmodium ovale*
(E) *Babesia microti*

87. Central nervous system involvement

88. Paroxysms of fever every third day

89. Splenectomy

90. Blackwater fever

Questions 91–96

Match the sputum examination results with the appropriate clinical setting.

(A) Pneumococcal pneumonia
(B) *Haemophilus influenzae* pneumonia
(C) *Staphylococcus aureus* pneumonia
(D) Tuberculosis
(E) Poor sputum specimen

91. Gram stain shows few epithelial cells, many neutrophils, gram-positive cocci in clusters

92. Gram stain shows few epithelial cells, many neutrophils, gram-positive cocci in pairs

93. Gram stain shows many epithelial cells, few neutrophils, gram-negative rods

94. Gram stain shows few epithelial cells, many neutrophils, gram-negative rods

95. Positive acid-fast stain

96. Positive quellung reaction

Questions 97–99

For each description below, select the drug combination with which it is most likely to be associated.

- (A) Chloramphenicol and phenytoin (Dilantin)
- (B) Isoniazid and rifampin
- (C) Tetracycline and antacids
- (D) Erythromycin and calcium supplements
- (E) Isoniazid and ethambutol

97. Decreased absorption of one drug due to the effect of the other

98. Increased risk of hepatotoxicity

99. Prolonged half-life of one drug due to a shared metabolic pathway with the other

Questions 100–104

Match the clinical presentation with the proper helminth.

- (A) *Ascaris lumbricoides*
- (B) *Necator americanus*
- (C) *Onchocerca volvulus*
- (D) *Trichinella spiralis*
- (E) *Strongyloides stercoralis*

100. Periorbital edema

101. Blindness

102. Gram-negative bacteremia

103. Iron-deficiency anemia

104. Intestinal obstruction

Questions 105–109

For each of the sexually transmitted diseases listed below, select the treatment of choice.

- (A) Penicillin
- (B) Doxycycline
- (C) Ceftriaxone plus doxycycline
- (D) Metronidazole
- (E) Acyclovir

105. Presumed gonococcal urethritis

106. Nongonococcal urethritis

107. Severe primary genital herpes

108. Trichomoniasis

109. Syphilis

Questions 110–113

Identify the antimicrobial agent associated with the adverse effects listed below.

- (A) Gentamicin
- (B) Imipenem
- (C) Tetracycline
- (D) Clindamycin
- (E) None of the above

110. Photosensitivity

111. Acute tubular necrosis

112. Progressive weakness in a patient with myasthenia gravis

113. Seizures

Questions 114–119

Match the clinical presentation with the proper helminth.

(A) *Trichuris trichiura*
(B) *Enterobius vermicularis*
(C) *Diphyllobothrium latum*
(D) *Taenia solium*
(E) *Taenia saginata*

114. Vitamin B_{12} deficiency

115. Cysticercosis

116. Perianal pruritus

117. Rectal prolapse

118. Illness following ingestion of raw fish

119. Illness following ingestion of raw pork

Infectious Disease

Answers

44.   The answer is D. *(Mandell, ed 3. pp 1465-1471.)* Rocky Mountain spotted fever is a disease transmitted by ticks and is the most common rickettsial infection in the U.S. More than 50 percent of cases occur in the South Atlantic region with a prevalence in the spring and summer. The infection is caused by the deposition of rickettsiae into the skin by ticks. A vasculitis of the small vessels is then produced, which may cause infarction in regions of the heart, brain, kidney, skin, and adrenal gland. Patients typically present with fever, chills, headache, and myalgias; a peripherally located, macular rash then appears on the third to fifth day of illness. Gastrointestinal symptoms such as nausea, vomiting, abdominal pain, or diarrhea may dominate the early presentation and suggest an acute surgical abdomen or gastroenteritis.

45.   The answer is B. *(Stein, ed 3. pp 1468-1472.)* Meningococci are gram-negative cocci or diplococci whose natural habitat is the nasopharynx; transmission from person to person is through inhalation of droplets of infected nasopharyngeal secretions. Meningococci may cause either epidemic or sporadic disease. While some people harbor meningococci for years, nasopharyngeal infection is usually transient. Between epidemics, 5 to 15 percent of the people in urban centers carry meningococci in the nasopharynx. In closed populations, the carrier state in close contacts approaches 80 percent. Nasopharyngeal carriage results in production of antibodies in 7 to 10 days. When invasive disease occurs after acquisition of carriage, it usually occurs before the development of specific antibodies. Because carriers, not patients, are the foci from which disease is spread, chemoprophylaxis should be administered to intimate contacts of sporadic cases of meningococcal disease. Rifampin in dosages of 600 mg every 12 h for 2 days for adults and 10 mg/kg body weight every 12 h for children will eradicate the carrier state temporarily and minimize the spread of meningococci.

46.   The answer is D. *(Stein, ed 3. pp 1432-1433.)* Toxic shock syndrome is a multiple organ system syndrome with a clinical picture of shock associated with fever and a characteristic sunburn-like rash with subsequent desquamation. Among the many laboratory abnormalities is hypocalcemia, which may be severe. This syndrome is caused by a toxin elaborated by *Staphylococcus aureus*; similar syndromes have less commonly been described in association with other bacteria, including group A streptococci.

47.   The answer is D. *(Stein, ed 3. pp 1573–1577.)* Meningitis or meningoencephalitis is the most common clinical manifestation of infection with the fungus *Cryptococcus neoformans.* The majority of patients are immunocompromised (i.e., they are receiving corticosteroids or immunosuppressive therapy or are infected with HIV), but about 35 percent have no identifiable predisposing immunologic defect. The diagnosis is confirmed by examination of the CSF. The India ink preparation of CSF will reveal budding yeast in about three-fourths of cases. Cryptococcal polysaccharide antigen is present in CSF in over 90 percent of cases; in most cases this antigen is also present in serum. Culture of CSF is usually positive; cultures of blood and urine are each positive for cryptococci in about one-fourth of patients.

48.   The answer is B. *(Mandell, ed 3. pp 2258–2265.)* Patients with Hodgkin's disease or AIDS or those receiving corticosteroid and cytotoxic agents all have in common a dysfunction of cellular immunity that leaves them particularly susceptible to infection with such pathogens as *Listeria monocytogenes, Legionella, Nocardia, Salmonella,* varicella-zoster virus, herpes simplex virus, *Toxoplasma gondii,* and *Strongyloides stercoralis,* as well as those listed in the question. Patients with humoral immune dysfunction, in contrast, lack opsonizing antibodies in their serum and therefore cannot adequately defend against encapsulated organisms such as *Haemophilus influenzae* and *Streptococcus pneumoniae.* Granulocytopenic patients and those with defective leukocyte phagocytic activity are prone to infection with *Candida, Aspergillus,* agents of mucormycosis, *Pseudomonas aeruginosa,* and certain other bacteria.

49.   The answer is B. *(Mandell, ed 3. p 2146.)* Human infection by the cercariae of one of the many nonhuman (bird) schistosomes is self-limited. On initial exposure, a mild dermatitis may not even be noticed. Sensitized persons develop more intense reactions, but the infection stops at this point without further progression because the organisms die in the dermis. The disease is commonly found in Canada and the northern United States.

50.   The answer is C. *(Mandell, ed 3. pp 1596–1597.)* Chagas' disease, caused by protozoa of the genus *Trypanosoma,* involves the development of both megaesophagus and megacolon with hypertrophy of smooth muscle. Unilateral conjunctivitis and edema of the eyelids—known as Romaña's sign—and myocarditis are also well recognized features of the disease.

51.   The answer is D. *(Mandell, ed 3. pp 479–487.)* Enteroviruses such as echovirus can cause maculopapular rashes and occasionally papulovesicular or petechial rashes. Other viruses and *Mycoplasma pneumoniae* are capable of provoking erythema multiforme eruptions. The location of the rash provides a useful diagnostic criterion. Maculopapular rashes in which there is a relative sparing of the palms and soles are generally caused by viruses. Eruptions associated with drug reactions, bacteria, *Mycoplasma,* and *Rickettsia* often feature a prominent palmar and plantar eruption. Transient "rose spots" may be seen over the abdomen in patients with typhoid fever. The maculopapular rash of roseola is usually transient, lasting only a few hours and rarely as long as 2 days.

52.   The answer is C. *(Stein, ed 3. pp 1577–1583.)* The occurrence of fever every 72 h is characteristic of early infection with *Plasmodium malariae,* or quartan malaria. This type of malaria can persist for many years with relapses as long as 20 years after infection. In falciparum malaria, however, a 48-h cycle is seen.

53.   The answer is C. *(Mandell, ed 3. pp 2110–2115.)* *Giardia lamblia* is a pear-shaped multiflagellated protozoan that parasitizes the human small intestine. The organism is transmitted by the fecal-oral route generally via contaminated water. The infection is found worldwide, especially in regions of poor sanitation and personal hygiene. Person-to-person transmission (e.g., between small children in day care centers, sexually active homosexual men) is now the second most commonly recognized mode of acquisition. *Giardia lamblia* is diagnosed in 3.9 percent of examined stools in the United States and is the most frequently identified intestinal parasite. Among sexually active homosexual men, cyst passage rates of 20 percent have been reported. However, the finding of *Giardia lamblia* in the stool from the patient described in the question is highly significant. The organisms frequently cause "traveler's diarrhea," characteristically beginning late in the course of travel and persisting for several weeks. Giardiasis is commonly associated with IgA deficiency, although IgA deficiency is not likely to be a factor in a previously well patient. Other conditions that predispose to giardiasis include gastrectomy and malnutrition. Irritability of the duodenal bulb often can be demonstrated radiographically. Rapid weight loss, along with lactase and disaccharidase deficiencies and general malabsorption, is commonly associated with giardiasis.

54.   The answer is A. *(Mandell, ed 3. pp 716–721.)* Although no evidence exists that prophylactic antibiotic therapy prevents endocarditis, prophylaxis is recommended for all procedures that may generate bacteremias. Following cardiac catheterization, blood cultures obtained from a distal vein rarely are positive. Thus, prophylactic antibiosis is not currently recommended for cardiac catheterization. Bacteremia occurs commonly following other procedures such as endoscopy, cystoscopy, sigmoidoscopy, and prostate surgery.

55.   The answer is D. *(Mandell, ed 3. pp 1291–1303.)* Rabies is caused by a bullet-shaped rhabdovirus. In the United States, dogs seldom are rabid. The animals that represent the most danger are wild skunks and bats; foxes also are possible carriers. Raccoons are responsible for an increasing number of cases in the mid-Atlantic states. The incubation period is variable, ranging from 4 days to many years, but is usually between 20 and 90 days. The incubation period is usually shorter with a bite to the head than with one to an extremity. In humans, only three definite recoveries from established infection have been reported. Nonimmunized animals that have bitten should be killed and their brains submitted for virus immunofluorescent antibody examination. A negative fluorescent test removes the need to treat the bite victim, either actively or passively.

56.   The answer is B. *(Mandell, ed 3. p 764. Wyngaarden, ed 18. pp 2195-2196.)* In active cases of herpes simplex encephalitis, it is rare to culture herpesvirus from the cerebrospinal fluid. Once found, the virus is easily grown; a biopsy specimen from an affected part of the brain, procured early in the course of the disease, is the best means of isolating it. When the index of suspicion is high, treatment with an agent such as acyclovir should be initiated early, even without confirmation of the diagnosis, because a favorable outcome correlates with early initiation of therapy.

57.   The answer is E (all). *(Mandell, ed 3. pp 2008-2017. Wilson, ed 12. pp 746-747.)* *Coccidioides immitis* has been found in certain semiarid and arid regions of Arizona, Texas, and New Mexico, as well as in Mexico and some parts of Central and South America. Persons entering these regions from nonendemic areas are liable to become infected with this organism, which causes fever, malaise, dry cough, chest pain, night sweats, and anorexia. Erythema nodosum or erythema multiforme and arthralgias may occur 3 days to 3 weeks after the onset of symptoms. The combination of erythema nodosum, arthralgias, and pneumonia represents the classic syndrome of valley fever (primary coccidioidomycosis). Headache and stiff neck occur much less commonly during primary infection. Risk of dissemination from a pulmonary focus is very high in Filipinos, blacks, and pregnant women.

58.   The answer is E (all). *(Mandell, ed 3. pp 370-393.)* Antiviral drugs are becoming increasingly available to treat a variety of viral infections. Unfortunately resistance to antiviral therapy has been observed with increasing frequency in the clinical setting, especially in immunocompromised patients receiving medication for prolonged periods. Antiviral resistance has been demonstrated in patients receiving acyclovir for herpes simplex infections, patients taking ganciclovir for CMV infections, and those on zidovudine (AZT) for HIV infection. Resistant virus has also been isolated from patients with acute influenza A infection after just several days' treatment with rimantadine (a drug related to amantadine). This would certainly argue for the prudent use of such agents.

59.   The answer is A (1, 2, 3). *(Wyngaarden, ed 18. pp 61-66.)* Adults over age 65 should receive the influenza vaccine on an annual basis. This vaccine is reformulated yearly to include the virus strains most likely to cause epidemics during the following winter. Pneumococcal vaccine should be administered once, although the duration of immunity is not known. Booster immunizations with Td (tetanus and diphtheria toxoids, adult type) should be performed every 10 years.

60.   The answer is B (1, 3). *(Mandell, ed 3. pp 1153–1159. Stein, ed 3. pp 1406–1407.)* Herpes zoster (shingles) usually is *unilateral* in distribution, causing a vesicular skin eruption that often halts abruptly at the midline of its dermatomal pattern. Despite a distinct association with Hodgkin's disease, zoster is not limited to patients with this disease. Frequently, pain along affected dermatomes persists for many weeks after the skin lesion has disappeared.

61.   The answer is A (1, 2, 3). *(Mandell, ed 3. p 713.)* Prosthetic arteriovenous fistulas suffer an infection rate higher than that noted for native-vessel fistulas. Most infections are caused by endogenous *S. aureus*, although *P. aeruginosa* is also a frequent isolate. Infections may occur at the time of implantation or through needle punctures at the time of dialysis; bacteremia is an uncommon source but is not an uncommon complication. Local erythema, pain, abscess formation, and hemorrhage from disruption of suture lines may occur, but an absence of remarkable local findings occurs in up to one-third of cases. Successful treatment of an infected arteriovenous fistula usually requires appropriate antibiotics plus surgery.

62.   The answer is E (all). *(Stein, ed 3. pp 1345–1347.)* Advice to travelers requires an understanding of the diseases likely to be encountered as a result of the journey in the setting of that particular patient's medical and immunization history. Not only should the physician give the traveler advice as to how to prevent certain illnesses (such as malaria and traveler's diarrhea) and administer any required immunizations, but this is also a good opportunity to review and update the patient's immunization record. Since the medical student is likely to have exposure to blood or other secretions of patients in a region where the carriage rate of hepatitis B is high, hepatitis B immunization would be recommended if it has not already been administered.

63.   The answer is A (1, 2, 3). *(Stein, ed 3. pp 1370–1371.)* Amantadine has been demonstrated to be effective in the treatment of uncomplicated influenza A illness when administered early in the course of infection. Amantadine will also prevent about 70 percent of influenza A illnesses if administered prophylactically. The influenza virus vaccine should not be administered to persons with allergy to eggs or egg products. Since vaccine is produced from inactivated viruses, it does not cause infection.

64.   The answer is D (4). *(Wilson, ed 12. pp 748–749, 2028.)* Patients who have cavernous sinus thrombosis with obstruction of the ophthalmic vein and involvement of cranial nerves III, IV, V, and VI are acutely ill and present characteristic eye findings of proptosis, chemosis, edema, and pain. Extension of the lesion through the intercavernous sinus to the contralateral sinus can be rapid. Although the commonest offending organism is *Staphylococcus aureus*, antibiotic therapy also should include coverage for *Proteus* and *Pseudomonas*. While mucormycosis and orbital cellulitis both enter the initial differential diagnosis of the patient discussed in the question, rapid spread of the lesion to the other eye in these disorders is uncommon.

65. The answer is C (2, 4). *(Mandell, ed 3. pp 1539–1550.)* The fatality rate in patients over the age of 12 with bacteremic pneumococcal pneumonia is about 20 percent. The rate is significantly higher in patients who are over the age of 50, especially patients with chronic disorders including cardiovascular disease, chronic bronchopulmonary and hepatic disease, diabetes, and renal insufficiency. The vaccine is recommended for all patients with sickle cell disease who are more than 2 years old. Unfortunately, the vaccine is of little use in children under the age of 2, who respond poorly to polysaccharide antigens, a circumstance that makes it difficult to protect them from many of the serious bacterial diseases that particularly affect this age group (e.g., *Haemophilus influenzae*, group B *Streptococcus, Meningococcus*). The vaccine is also recommended for adults with chronic cardiovascular or pulmonary disease and adults with splenic dysfunction or other immune suppression, including persons with alcoholism, cirrhosis, renal failure, and CSF leaks.

66. The answer is B (1, 3). *(Mandell, ed 3. p 2325. Stein, ed 3. pp 1461–1465.)* Tetanus toxin, produced by *Clostridium tetani*, causes prolonged muscle spasms of flexor and extensor muscle groups. The masseter and respiratory muscles may be involved and produce lockjaw and respiratory paralysis, respectively. Patients with any type of wound must be considered for tetanus prophylaxis and adequate debridement of the wound. Adults are considered adequately immunized if they have completed a three-dose primary immunization series within 10 years, or if they have received such a series earlier and been given a booster within 10 years. Inadequately immunized adults should receive a booster of Td (tetanus and diphtheria toxoids, adult type) if they completed the primary series, or a series of boosters if they did not. Hyperimmune antitetanus gamma globulin should be given only to patients who either have tetanus or have tetanus-prone wounds and have received either no previous immunization or only a single dose. The pertussis vaccine is usually not recommended for adults because the risk of infection seems to be lower and because vaccine reactions may be more frequent.

67. The answer is C (2, 4). *(Mandell, ed 3. pp 2145–2149.)* Schistosomes are endemic to Puerto Rico, Brazil, the Middle East, and the Philippines and require an appropriate snail intermediate host, which is absent in the U.S., for transmission. The patient in the question, then, is not a threat for spreading infection. Unlike *S. mansoni* and *S. japonicum*, which cause hepatomegaly and diarrhea, *S. haematobium* affects the ureters and bladder, where granulomatous reactions to the eggs occur and may lead to urinary obstruction. Praziquantel is a broad-spectrum anti-helminthic agent and is the drug of choice for all human schistosome species; it is well tolerated and only occasionally causes fever, headache, and abdominal discomfort. Other agents effective against schistosomes include metrifonate, which is effective against *S. haematobium*, and oxamniquine, which is effective against *S. mansoni*.

68.   The answer is C (2, 4). *(Stein, ed 3. pp 1447-1448.)* *Streptococcus bovis* is a nonenterococcal group D streptococcus that is susceptible to penicillin. Between 5 and 10 percent of normal adults will have *S. bovis* in their stools. Because of an association between *S. bovis* endocarditis and occult colonic neoplasms, persons diagnosed with this infection should undergo colonoscopy or barium enema or both. Unlike infection with group A streptococci, infection with group D streptococci is not associated with sequelae such as rheumatic fever.

69.   The answer is E (all). *(Wyngaarden, ed 18. pp 1838-1840.)* *Histoplasma capsulatum* is an airborne microorganism causing primary infection of the lung. Lymphatic spread to regional lymph nodes and hematogenous spread to the liver and spleen are common. Infection in all these sites is suppressed by the immune response. A small number of affected patients may suffer relapse associated with hepatosplenomegaly and fever. This type of chronic disseminated histoplasmosis may be mistaken for a lymphoma. Disseminated infection may involve the adrenals, endocardium, pericardium, oropharynx, and larynx, as well as the meninges. Chronic pulmonary histoplasmosis resembles chronic pulmonary tuberculosis and may be associated with cavities.

70.   The answer is E (all). *(Chow, Rev Infect Dis 7:287-313, 1985.)* In terms of maternal toxicity, both erythromycin estolate and tetracycline are associated with hepatotoxicity, trimethoprim-sulfamethoxazole with vasculitis, and chloramphenicol with bone marrow aplasia. No known fetal damage occurs as a result of erythromycin estolate administration. In contrast, chloramphenicol is associated with the gray baby syndrome; tetracycline, because it avidly binds to developing bone, with inhibition of bone growth; and trimethoprim-sulfamethoxazole with various congenital anomalies. Essentially all antibiotics are excreted in breast milk, which is an important concern especially in relation to premature infants and those with hereditary enzyme defects.

71.   The answer is E (all). *(Wilson, ed 12. pp 581-582.)* A relatively common complication of antibiotic therapy is diarrhea. The diarrhea may result from changes in microbial flora or production of a toxin produced by *Clostridium difficile*. Colonoscopic examination may reveal colitis and pseudomembranes (pseudomembranous colitis). Whereas it was previously believed that only clindamycin caused pseudomembranous colitis, it has more recently been appreciated that this complication may result from virtually any antibiotic.

72–76. The answers are: 72-A, 73-C, 74-D, 75-B, 76-E. *(Mandell, ed 3. pp 893–905.)* The clinical history is helpful in identifying the specific bacterial agent responsible for food poisoning. The symptoms and, when known, the incubation period and type of offending food can provide helpful clues. In general, disease mediated by preformed toxins has a shorter incubation period (e.g., *Staphylococcus aureus*, 1 to 6 h) than disease due to tissue invasion. *Clostridium perfringens* produces its toxin in vivo after ingestion. Fever is uncommon in illness caused by these toxins. Lower intestinal symptoms predominate with illness from *Clostridium*-contaminated food, whereas upper intestinal symptoms predominate with illness from staphylococcus-contaminated food.

Ingestion of bacteria with subsequent invasion of the intestinal mucosa has been associated with *Shigella sonnei* and other *Shigella* species, *Salmonella* species, *Vibrio parahaemolyticus,* and *Yersinia enterocolitica.* Illness caused by these microorganisms in food is generally associated with fever, abdominal pain, and diarrhea. Severe cramps and bloody diarrhea are associated with the *Shigella* infections. *Vibrio parahaemolyticus* has been associated with contaminated crabs caught in the Chesapeake Bay, and high salt concentrations in culture media are required to isolate this microorganism. *Yersinia enterocolitica,* which commonly causes infection in northern Europe, has also been identified in the United States. Symptoms of infection with this organism may mimic appendicitis.

77–81. The answers are: 77-E, 78-D, 79-C, 80-B, 81-A. *(Mandell, ed 3. pp 1261, 1354–1355, 1375–1376. Wilson, ed 12. pp 686–689, 705–707, 709–711, 715–716, 717–720.)* Although salivary adenitis is the most prominent feature of the communicable disease of viral-origin mumps, it is not uncommon to have involvement of the gonads, meninges, and pancreas. Males who develop mumps after the age of puberty have a 20 to 35 percent chance of developing a painful orchitis. Central nervous system involvement is common but usually mild, with 50 percent of cases having an increase in lymphocytes detectable in the CSF. Myocarditis, thrombocytopenic purpura, and polyarthritis may also occur as complications of this disease. An inflammatory change in the pancreas, however, is a potentially serious problem; symptoms consist of abdominal discomfort and a gastroenteritis-like illness.

Although a polyneuritis and a transverse myelitis have been described, the most common manifestation of CNS infection with varicella is acute cerebellar ataxia. While chickenpox is usually a benign illness in children, other complications such as myocarditis, iritis, nephritis, orchitis, and hepatitis may occur. Pneumonitis occurs more commonly in adults than children.

It can be difficult to distinguish between the vesicular lesions of smallpox and chickenpox. Classically, however, a history of a rash with vesicles developing over a few hours would be typical of a chickenpox infection; vesiculation developing over a period of days is the rule in smallpox. While fever is characteristic of the prodrome of smallpox, it subsides prior to focal eruptions. Lesions of smallpox are typically all at the same stage of development, in contrast to the various stages seen in a patient with chickenpox. Preparations of vesicular fluid under electron microscopy show characteristic brick-shaped particles with poxvirus. A more readily available test, the Tzanck smear, performed by scraping the base of the lesion, should reveal multinucleated giant cells microscopically in a patient with chickenpox.

Humoral immunity appears to be very important in the recovery from enteroviral infections. One of the most common complications for patients with sex-linked or acquired agammaglobulinemia is a chronic central nervous system infection with an echovirus. In the absence of the ability to produce antibodies, this virus spreads rapidly and usually produces a fatal illness. The administration of intravenous preparations of gamma globulin intraventricularly has controlled this serious complication of immune deficiency in some patients.

It may take from 9 to 11 days for the first symptoms of measles to develop after exposure. Malaise, irritability, and a high fever often associated with conjunctivitis with prominent tearing are common symptoms. This prodromal syndrome may last from 3 days to a week before the characteristic rash of measles develops. One or two days before the onset of the rash, characteristic Koplik's spots—small, red, irregular lesions with blue-white centers—may be visible on the mucous membranes and occasionally on the conjunctiva. Classically, the measles rash will begin on the forehead and spread downward and the Koplik's spots will rapidly resolve.

82–86. The answers are: 82-A, 83-D, 84-B, 85-E, 86-C. *(Wyngaarden, ed 18. pp 1799–1808.)* The number of opportunistic infections occurring in patients with AIDS continues to grow. Pneumonia due to *Pneumocystis carinii* was among the first recognized manifestations of AIDS. The chest radiograph typically shows a diffuse bilateral interstitial pattern, but other patterns including a normal radiograph may occur. *Pneumocystis* infection may also occur at extrapulmonary sites.

Cytomegalovirus (CMV) is a frequent disseminated pathogen causing retinitis leading to blindness. CMV may also cause pneumonitis, adrenalitis, and hepatitis, as well as colitis with significant diarrhea.

The protozoa *Cryptosporidium* may cause a chronic diarrhea leading to malabsorption and wasting. It can be diagnosed by direct examination of the stool with special concentration or staining techniques or both.

Salmonella infections have been recognized with increased frequency in patients with HIV. These patients are typically bacteremic and develop bacteremic relapse; they do not usually present with a diarrheal illness.

Patients who present with seizures warrant an evaluation for toxoplasmosis. CNS lymphoma and certain other infections may also cause seizures.

87-90.   The answers are: 87-C, 88-B, 89-E, 90-C. *(Stein, ed 3. pp 1577-1583.)* Although slow but definite progress is being made toward the development of a vaccine to prevent malaria, attempts in developing countries to eradicate the *Anopheles* mosquito or its breeding grounds have failed. Malaria is on the increase throughout the tropics, and eradication attempts appear to have resulted in the survival of more hardy strains of plasmodia. In a number of areas they have become resistant to the simple antimalarial drugs. Approximately 1000 cases a year are reported in the United States, mainly in patients who become infected while abroad. Of the four species of plasmodia that cause malaria, *P. falciparum* is the most important as it causes most of the clinical cases of malaria in the world and is associated with a large number of complications. Multiple infections of single red blood cells occur and organisms have the capacity to block the microcirculation in various organs. Cerebral involvement is common and frequently fatal in children. Seizures, focal disorders, delirium, and coma may occur. Blackwater fever occurs in association with malaria—particularly and perhaps only with falciparum malaria. For all forms of malaria the rupture of parasitized red cells with subsequent reinvasion of new cells is associated with paroxysms of chills and fever. Whereas *P. vivax* and *P. ovale* infections tend to cause alternate-day fevers, infections with *P. malariae* are associated with spiking temperatures every 72 h (quartan malaria).

Babesiosis is a disease similar to malaria and also caused by a protozoan parasite that lives inside red blood cells. Babesiosis has been reported to be endemic on Nantucket Island but has also been found on other islands off the Massachusetts coast and other Atlantic coast states, as well as Georgia, Wisconsin, Minnesota, California, and Mexico. Although the disease can be mild, it is particularly serious in patients who have previously undergone splenectomy for an unrelated condition. In such patients very high fevers, drenching sweats, chills, lethargy, myalgias, arthralgias, and psychiatric disturbances are common. As many as 40 percent of the red cells may be infected. Orally administered quinine in combination with parenteral clindamycin constitutes the treatment of choice for life-threatening disease.

91-96.   The answers are: 91-C, 92-A, 93-E, 94-B, 95-D, 96-A. *(Stein, ed 3. p 1266.)* Examination of a freshly collected sputum specimen is crucial to the early bacteriologic diagnosis of pneumonia and aids greatly in selection of initial antibiotic therapy. An adequate specimen should not be contaminated by oropharyngeal flora, as would be suggested by the presence of many squamous epithelial cells. Knowledge of the appropriate microscopic morphology allows for identification of pathogens: staphylococci, gram-positive cocci in clusters; pneumococci, gram-positive cocci in pairs; *H. influenzae*, small gram-negative rods. The presence of pneumococci can be confirmed by a positive quellung test (a refractory halo around each organism after the addition of serum containing antibodies to the capsular polysaccharide). Tuberculosis may be suggested by a positive acid-fast stain.

97-99.   The answers are: 97-C, 98-B, 99-A. *(Mandell, ed 3. p 292. Wyngaarden, ed 18. p 124.)* Combinations of drugs may have unexpected effects. The gastrointestinal absorption of one of two combined drugs may be reduced, as occurs when tetracycline is combined with antacids.

Increased toxic effects from one or both drugs also may result from combined drug therapy, as in rifampin with isoniazid (increased hepatotoxicity) and aminoglycosides with skeletal muscle relaxants (respiratory paralysis).

Finally, the half-life of one of the two drugs may be prolonged if they share a common metabolic pathway. In this manner, chloramphenicol prolongs the half-life of phenytoin (Dilantin), warfarin (Coumadin), and tolbutamide; isoniazid prolongs the half-life of phenytoin; and sulfonamides prolong the half-life of tolbutamide.

100-104.   The answers are: 100-D, 101-C, 102-E, 103-B, 104-A. *(Stein, ed 3. pp 1605-1613.)* *Trichinella spiralis* is the cause of trichinosis. Humans become infected after eating larvae in raw or undercooked meat. The typical presentation of periorbital edema, myalgias, petechial hemorrhages, and eosinophilia occurs after an incubation period of 1 to 2 weeks.

Onchocerca volvulus is a major cause of blindness worldwide. The disease onchocerciasis is also known as river blindness because it is caused by the bite of an infected blackfly that breeds in rivers and streams.

Strongyloides stercoralis causes a potentially fatal disseminated infection (hyperinfection) in immunocompromised patients. Such patients may present with gram-negative bacteremia and multiple organ system involvement. This diagnosis should be excluded before a patient with eosinophilia is begun on immunosuppressive therapy.

Patients with *Ascaris lumbricoides* infection may present with intestinal or biliary obstruction.

Iron-deficiency anemia may be detected in asymptomatic persons infected with hookworm (*Necator americanus* or *Ancylostoma duodenale*).

105-109.   The answers are: 105-C, 106-B, 107-E, 108-D, 109-A. *(Centers for Disease Control, MMWR 38(5-8): 1-43, 1989.)* Treatment of gonococcal infections in the 1990s should be guided by the increasing frequency of antibiotic-resistant *Neisseria gonorrhoeae* and high frequency of coinfection with *Chlamydia trachomatis*. Because of the increased frequency of resistance to penicillin and tetracyclines, ceftriaxone is recommended as the treatment of choice. Doxycycline is added to treat chlamydial and other causes of nongonococcal urethritis.

First episodes of genital herpes may be particularly severe. Oral acyclovir will accelerate the healing but will not reduce the risk of recurrence once the drug is stopped.

Trichomoniasis is usually diagnosed by a wet preparation microscopic examination or by culture. Both the patient and sexual partner should be treated with metronidazole.

Penicillin remains the drug of choice for treatment of syphilis. The route of administration and duration of therapy depend on the stage of disease and presence of CNS involvement and may also be influenced by the HIV-serostatus of the patient.

110–113. The answers are: 110-C, 111-A, 112-A, 113-B. *(Stein, ed 3. pp 1210–1217, 1456–1458.)* The tetracyclines are associated with photosensitization, and patients taking these antibiotics should be warned about exposure to the sun.

Imipenem, a carbapenem, may cause central nervous system toxicity such as seizures, especially when administered at high dosages.

The major toxicity of gentamicin, an aminoglycoside, is acute tubular necrosis; thus, drug levels should be closely monitored. The aminoglycosides may be ototoxic, with effects on vestibular or auditory function or both. This class of drugs can also produce neuromuscular blockade, especially when administered with concomitant neuromuscular blocking agents or to patients with impairment of neuromuscular transmission, such as myasthenia gravis.

114–119. The answers are: 114-C, 115-D, 116-B, 117-A, 118-C, 119-D. *(Stein, ed 3. pp 1602–1615.)* The intestinal worms, for the most part, produce disease localized to or resulting from their presence in the gastrointestinal tract. A notable exception occurs with the ingestion of eggs from the pork tapeworm, *Taenia solium.* Larval migration and dissemination throughout the body occur with the formation of fluid-filled cysts. This stage of disease, cysticercosis, can involve almost any tissue in the body, including the central nervous system. Unlike the other helminth infections, such as *Taenia saginata* (beef tapeworm) infection, which are not associated with tissue migration, eosinophilia does occur in cysticercosis and may be very pronounced in association with cyst degeneration.

Trichuris trichiura, the whipworm, may produce rectal prolapse and diarrhea, although most infected patients are asymptomatic.

The adult pinworm, *Enterobius vermicularis,* resides in the intestines. The female worm, after migrating to the rectum at night, deposits her ova on the perirectal mucosa. These eggs are irritative and lead to perianal pruritus.

The fish tapeworm, *Diphyllobothrium latum,* has an affinity for vitamin B_{12} and may lead to megaloblastic anemia.

Rheumatology

DIRECTIONS: Each question below contains five suggested responses. Select the **one best** response to each question.

120. A 55-year-old man awakens with excruciating pain in the first metatarsophalangeal joint of his right foot. His physician identifies needle-shaped, negatively birefringent crystals in synovial fluid aspirated from the affected joint. The most desirable therapy for this patient would be

(A) allopurinol, 300 mg
(B) colchicine, 3 mg twice a day
(C) sulfinpyrazone, 400 mg daily
(D) indomethacin, 200 mg daily in divided doses
(E) salicylate, 3800 mg daily in divided doses

121. Ankylosing spondylitis is associated with all the following features EXCEPT

(A) peripheral arthritis
(B) abnormalities of cardiac conduction
(C) uveitis
(D) pulmonary fibrosis
(E) Sjögren's syndrome

122. A 25-year-old man who admits to frequent self-administration of intravenous drugs presents at an emergency room with right knee pain and swelling of 24 h duration. The pain is moderately severe with movement. He gives a 1-week history of pain and swelling in the fingers of both hands and a 2-day history of urticaria. He has a chronic cough. The patient has a temperature of 37.8°C (100°F) and limitation of flexion at the metacarpophalangeal and proximal interphalangeal joints of both hands. A small effusion is noted in the right knee. A flat, slightly pruritic erythematous rash is noted on his arms and legs. The most likely diagnosis of this man's disorder would be

(A) gonococcal arthritis
(B) rheumatoid arthritis
(C) rheumatoid arthritis complicated by a septic arthritis
(D) tuberculous arthritis
(E) viral hepatitis complicated by arthritis

123. Deposition of calcium pyrophosphate dihydrate crystals may cause local damage. Such crystals may cause all the following EXCEPT

(A) acute monarticular inflammation
(B) pseudorheumatoid disease
(C) pseudo-osteoarthritis
(D) asymptomatic chondrocalcinosis
(E) pseudoankylosing spondylitis

124. A 65-year-old woman who has a 12-year history of symmetrical polyarthritis is admitted to the hospital. Physical examination reveals splenomegaly, ulcerations over the anterior shins, and synovitis of the wrists, shoulders, and knees. Splenomegaly, but no hepatomegaly, is noted. Laboratory values demonstrate a white blood cell count of $2500/mm^3$ and a rheumatoid factor titer of 1:4096. This patient's white blood cell differential count is likely to reveal

(A) pancytopenia
(B) lymphopenia
(C) granulocytopenia
(D) lymphocytosis
(E) basophilia

125. Arthritis of the temporomandibular joint may be caused by all the following diseases EXCEPT

(A) gout
(B) Lyme disease
(C) adult rheumatoid arthritis
(D) juvenile rheumatoid arthritis
(E) osteoarthritis

126. A 17-year-old black girl with a diagnosis of systemic lupus erythematosus (SLE) is referred to you for further evaluation. Among the problems you might expect her to experience would be all the following EXCEPT

(A) Coombs-positive hemolytic anemia
(B) proteinuria
(C) seizures or psychotic episodes or both
(D) deforming arthritis
(E) fever, fatigue, or weight loss, or all three

127. A 36-year-old white woman complains of painful joints and morning stiffness that has developed over the last 6 months. Factors suggesting the diagnosis of rheumatoid arthritis include all the following EXCEPT

(A) hot, red, swollen, and tender knees, wrists, and hands in a bilaterally symmetrical distribution
(B) the presence of a firm nodule in the olecranon bursa
(C) a family history of rheumatoid arthritis
(D) inflammation of distal interphalangeal joints
(E) wasting of dorsal interosseous muscle

128. All the following statements about scleroderma are correct EXCEPT that

(A) skin telangiectasias are frequent and may be numerous
(B) weakness and atrophy of the distal muscle groups usually occur
(C) pulmonary interstitial fibrosis independent of pulmonary hypertension is common in advanced disease
(D) stricture of the large bowel secondary to fibrosis in the wall of the intestine may lead to intestinal obstruction
(E) the patient with CREST syndrome rarely has cardiac involvement

DIRECTIONS: Each question below contains four suggested responses of which **one or more** is correct. Select

A	if	**1, 2, and 3**	are correct
B	if	**1 and 3**	are correct
C	if	**2 and 4**	are correct
D	if	**4**	is correct
E	if	**1, 2, 3, and 4**	are correct

129. Correct statements about psoriatic arthritis include which of the following?

(1) Arthritis occurs in 20 to 25 percent of patients with psoriasis
(2) HLA–B27 is strongly associated with sacroiliitis and spondylitis, but not peripheral arthritis, in patients with psoriatic arthritis
(3) Seventy percent of patients with psoriatic arthritis have seronegative symmetrical polyarthritis
(4) The flexor tendon sheaths in the fingers are often inflamed, producing "sausage" digits

130. Local causes of shoulder pain include bursitis and tendinitis. True statements about these disorders include which of the following?

(1) Rheumatoid arthritis may be a predisposing factor in bursitis
(2) Of the rotator cuff muscles, the most commonly affected by tendinitis is the supraspinatus
(3) A crystal-induced cause of shoulder pain is the "Milwaukee shoulder syndrome," caused by calcium hydroxyapatite crystals
(4) Following rotator cuff inflammation, a "frozen shoulder," or adhesive capsulitis, may occur, with near universal permanent disability

131. Charcot's joints are associated with which of the following conditions?

(1) Syringomyelia
(2) Diabetes mellitus
(3) Syphilis
(4) Ankylosing spondylitis

132. Correct statements about the etiology and pathogenesis of osteoarthritis include which of the following?

(1) Osteoarthritic cartilage undergoes increased metabolic activity and increased cell division, indicating that increased degradation and increased synthesis of cartilage matrix occur concurrently
(2) Osteoarthritis of the wrists, elbows, and shoulders is uncommon but may be found in persons subjected to occupational trauma
(3) Extensive osteoarthritis may be found late in the course of acromegaly
(4) Routine laboratory tests show no abnormalities in osteoarthritis

133. Sjögren's syndrome is associated with which of the following diseases?

(1) Scleroderma
(2) Polymyositis
(3) Systemic lupus erythematosus
(4) Rheumatoid arthritis

SUMMARY OF DIRECTIONS

A	B	C	D	E
1, 2, 3	1, 3	2, 4	4	All are
only	only	only	only	correct

134. A 17-year-old white male high school student seeks medical advice because of recurrent low back pain and stiffness that last for a few days after each football game and practice. No morning stiffness is noted. The patient is otherwise healthy and has no family history of joint problems and no abnormal physical findings. Radiographic examination of his spine and sacroiliac joint reveals no abnormalities. Serologic studies are not helpful and the patient's erythrocyte sedimentation rate is 13 mm/h (Westergren method). However, the patient is found to have the histocompatibility antigen HLA–B27 on his leukocytes. With this information, the physician can now advise the patient that

(1) it would be advisable to have an x-ray examination of his large bowel
(2) he should have a slitlamp examination of his eyes
(3) he should have gold therapy for the next year while his physician observes him closely for signs of developing spondylitis
(4) he has a 25 percent chance of developing significant spondylitis

135. Osteoarthritis is correctly characterized by which of the following statements?

(1) It has an approximately equal incidence in men and women
(2) It is usually associated with osteoporosis
(3) It may be initiated by acute trauma to a joint
(4) It is usually associated with white blood cell counts greater than 10,000/mm^3 in synovial fluid

136. Correct statements about Lyme disease include which of the following?

(1) The disease is caused by a spirochete that is spread by the *Ixodes dammini* tick
(2) The disease has been found to be the cause of arthritis on both the east and west coasts of the United States and in Australia and Europe
(3) Tetracycline is an effective antibiotic for newly diagnosed patients as it minimizes complications
(4) Lyme disease affects many body systems, and severe degrees of heart block may develop

137. The peripheral arthritis associated with inflammatory bowel disease is characterized by which of the following statements?

(1) It may be deforming
(2) It is associated with antinuclear antibody (ANA)
(3) It is more common in ulcerative colitis than in Crohn's disease
(4) It is often migratory

DIRECTIONS: Each group of questions below consists of lettered headings followed by a set of numbered items. For each numbered item select the **one** lettered heading with which it is **most** closely associated. Each lettered heading may be used **once, more than once, or not at all.**

Questions 138–142

For each condition select the drug with which it is closely associated.

(A) Acetylsalicylic acid (aspirin)
(B) Gold
(C) Prednisone
(D) Chloroquine
(E) None of the above

138. Gastrointestinal bleeding

139. Osteoporosis

140. Retinopathy

141. Proteinuria

142. Stomatitis

Questions 143–147

Match each description with the appropriate disease.

(A) Polyarteritis nodosa
(B) Wegener's granulomatosis
(C) Giant cell arteritis
(D) Multiple cholesterol embolization syndrome
(E) Takayasu's arteritis

143. Involvement of the upper and lower respiratory tracts; a cause of glomerulonephritis

144. Ecchymoses and necrosis in extremities in elderly patients

145. Inflammation of small- to medium-size muscular arteries, which may cause kidney, heart, liver, gastrointestinal, and muscular damage

146. Patients above the age of 55, who may experience fever, weight loss, scalp pain, headache, and visual changes

147. Inflammation of the aorta and its branches in young women; also known as "pulseless disease"

DIRECTIONS: The group of questions below consists of four lettered headings followed by a set of numbered items. For each numbered item select

A	if the item is associated with	(A) **only**
B	if the item is associated with	(B) **only**
C	if the item is associated with	**both** (A) and (B)
D	if the item is associated with	**neither** (A) nor (B)

Each lettered heading may be used **once, more than once, or not at all.**

Questions 148–152

(A) Gonococcal arthritis
(B) Reiter's syndrome
(C) Both
(D) Neither

148. Uveitis

149. Balanitis

150. Arthritis involving predominantly joints of the upper extremities

151. Six to eight percent of patients HLA-B27-positive

152. Stomatitis

Rheumatology
Answers

120. The answer is D. *(Wilson, ed 12. pp 1834–1841.)* Appropriate therapy of acute gouty arthritis can be divided into two phases. In the first phase, the acute gouty inflammation is controlled by anti-inflammatory agents or by giving colchicine, orally or intravenously. In the second phase, the serum urate level is lowered by uricosuric agents or drugs designed to inhibit the development of uric acid. Traditionally, acute gouty inflammation has been controlled by giving colchicine on an hourly basis until a therapeutic response occurs. However, as many as 80 percent of gout patients cannot achieve satisfactory therapeutic levels with colchicine because of the toxicity of the drug. Certainly, colchicine 3 mg twice a day would be too high a dose, although 2 mg given intravenously may give very good results. Anti-inflammatory drugs such as indomethacin or phenylbutazone have been found to be as effective as colchicine and to have fewer of the gastrointestinal side effects frequently associated with colchicine. Sulfinpyrazone and probenecid, both uricosuric agents, are not effective in acute flare. Allopurinol, a xanthine oxidase inhibitor, and the uricosuric agents probenecid and sulfinpyrazone effectively reverse hyperuricemia, but do not relieve inflammation associated with acute attacks of gouty arthritis. Allopurinol would be inappropriate therapy during an acute flare, in that this drug can precipitate further activity of gout.

121. The answer is E. *(Wilson, ed 12. pp 1451–1455.)* Ankylosing spondylitis, an inflammation of the spine, also involves the hip, shoulder, and, in 25 percent of patients, the peripheral joints. It is often associated with aortic regurgitation, conduction abnormalities that may require pacemaker therapy, acute anterior uveitis in 30 percent of patients, and, in long-standing disease, bilateral pulmonary fibrosis of the upper lobe. HLA-B27 is found in the vast majority of patients; the linkage is weaker in nonwhite persons. Ankylosing spondylitis must be differentiated from other diseases associated with spondylitis, such as inflammatory bowel disease, psoriatic arthritis, and Reiter's syndrome. The clinical course is characterized by remissions and exacerbations, although a persistently progressive course may occur. Symptomatic relief may be achieved using nonsteroidal anti-inflammatory drugs. Pain often disappears after total ankylosis of the joint occurs. The uveitis is treated with intraocular steroids. The progression of the disease is not halted, however, by any of these measures. Sjögren's syndrome is not seen in ankylosing spondylitis.

122. The answer is E. *(Wilson, ed 12. pp 545–547, 596–599, 1331, 1437–1443, 1459–1460.)* Arthritis is a relatively common manifestation of hepatitis B virus infection, as is the occurrence of urticaria in the prodromal phase. Clinically detectable jaundice may not develop for a few days or even weeks after the onset of a severe arthritis, which tends to be migratory and involves both small and large joints. As the involvement in the hands is frequently symmetrical, it is easily confused with rheumatoid arthritis. The arthritis may be accompanied by a rash. Suspicion of a hepatitis-induced arthritis can be confirmed by the detection of abnormal liver functions, especially elevated liver enzymes, while hepatitis B virus antigen, and perhaps antibody, will be detected in the serum and joint fluid. Low complement levels in the synovial fluid indicate active antigen-antibody complex deposition. Permanent joint damage may develop rapidly as a complication of septic arthritis. Early diagnosis with appropriate management of the arthritis is essential if this complication is to be avoided. Infectious arthritis can arise from viral, bacterial, and mycotic infections and although the diagnosis relies heavily on examination and culture of the joint fluid, these observations may not be immediately helpful. *Haemophilus influenzae*, which frequently causes meningitis in children, is most often responsible for a septic arthritis in childhood. Septic arthritis due to *Staphylococcus aureus* is now frequently encountered in drug-addicted persons who administer their drugs by an intravenous route. Gonococcal arthritis, which may present as a migratory polyarthralgia or tenosynovitis, remains a disease of sexually active persons; women are particularly prone to develop a gonococcal bacteremia at the time of menstruation with seeding of their joints. Bilateral and symmetrical synovial thickening of the joints of the hands and wrists is unusual in septic arthritis. Pustular skin rash may be found in gonococcal arthritis. Rheumatoid arthritis is usually an insidious process and is more common in women than men. Usually it is not associated with a rash, although Still's disease occurring in adults features a generalized rash. Patients with rheumatoid arthritis who present with sudden localized pain and swelling in a single joint should be carefully evaluated for a septic complication of their underlying joint disease; underlying joint disease increases susceptibility to secondary septic involvement of a joint space. Bacterial sepsis usually presents with acute onset of joint inflammation, severe splinting, and restriction of movement. Tuberculous arthritis, although now very rare, is more likely to arise in children than adults. Arthritis is not acute in onset and develops slowly, with spine, hips, and knees being particularly susceptible. Symmetrical disease of the hands is rare in tuberculosis, while the thickened synovium found in this condition has a characteristic boggy or doughy feeling.

123. The answer is E. *(Wilson, ed 12. pp 1480, 1826, 1834–1841, 1904.)* Calcium pyrophosphate dihydrate (CPPD) deposition disease may produce an asymptomatic calcification in cartilages (especially the knees, symphysis pubis, and triangular ligament of the wrists) called chondrocalcinosis. This is relatively common in older persons and by itself causes no damage. Monarticular inflammation, resembling a flare of gout and called "pseudogout," can be seen in CPPD deposition and be diagnosed by synovial fluid analysis. Clinically, pseudogout is identical to gout. A pattern of joint disease resembling rheumatoid arthritis, called pseudo-rheumatoid arthritis, may occur. Inflammation is present by history and on clinical examination, but these patients do not have circulating rheumatoid factor and their joints show a pattern of destruction more like extensive osteoarthritis than the classic pattern of rheumatoid arthritis. CPPD deposition disease can be associated with extensive osteoarthritic changes that appear to be virtually identical to those of osteoarthritis on x-ray, but occur in an atypical distribution, e.g., affecting the metacarpophalangeal joints, wrists, elbows, shoulders, and ankles. When this clinical picture occurs, the clinician should suspect CPPD deposition disease and consider the metabolic causes of CPPD deposition disease, which include hyperparathyroidism and hemochromatosis, most notably. The clinical course of pseudo-rheumatoid arthritis and pseudo-osteoarthritis may be punctuated by flares of pseudogout. CPPD deposition disease is not associated with spine disease, or anything resembling ankylosing spondylitis.

124.   The answer is C. *(Wilson, ed 12. pp 357–359, 1439.)* Felty's syndrome consists of a triad of rheumatoid arthritis, splenomegaly, and leukopenia. In contrast to the lymphopenia observed in patients who have systemic lupus erythematosus, the leukopenia of Felty's syndrome is related to a reduction in the number of circulating polymorphonuclear leukocytes. The mechanism of the granulocytopenia is poorly understood. Felty's syndrome tends to occur in people who have had active rheumatoid arthritis for a prolonged period. These patients commonly have other systemic features of rheumatoid disease such as nodules, skin ulcerations, the sicca complex, peripheral sensory and motor neuropathy, and arteritic lesions.

125.   The answer is A. *(Wilson, ed 12. pp 148, 667–669.)* Temporomandibular joint involvement is a classic feature of juvenile rheumatoid arthritis and, when present prior to closure of the epiphysis of the mandible, may result in micrognathia. Adult rheumatoid arthritis frequently causes temporomandibular joint symptoms. Lyme disease frequently affects the temporomandibular joint, often early in the course of the disease (stage I). Osteoarthritis can affect the joint in a smaller percentage of cases. Gout does not affect this particular joint.

126.   The answer is D. *(Wilson, ed 12. pp 1432–1437.)* Hematologic disease is frequent in SLE, with lymphopenia, leukopenia, anemia, or thrombocytopenia serving as one of the American College of Rheumatology criteria for the diagnosis of SLE. Other criteria include proteinuria or cellular casts (there are a number of different histologic patterns on kidney biopsy), neurologic disease (seizures or psychosis or both; peripheral neuropathy and organic brain syndromes also occur, but are not on the criteria list), cardiopulmonary disease (pleurisy and pericarditis—the old name for SLE was *polyserositis*), cutaneous lesions (malar rash in a "butterfly" distribution, discoid lesions, photosensitivity rash, and oral ulcers are each a separate criterion), and arthritis. The arthritis of SLE is typically a nonerosive, nondeforming polyarthritis; the hand deformities, rarely seen, are due to ligamentous laxity at the metacarpophalangeal joints that causes pseudosubluxation—so-called Jaccoud's arthritis. Fever, fatigue, malaise, anorexia, nausea, and weight loss are frequent systemic manifestations of SLE and often quite difficult to treat. SLE is more common in people of African, Asian, and Hispanic descent than in whites in the U.S.; 90 percent of all cases occur in women. Patients with SLE usually have antinuclear antibodies in their serum (although this test is *not* specific for SLE), as well as an ever-increasing number of other autoantibodies, including antibodies binding to neurons, lymphocytes, erythrocytes, platelets, and many cellular and nuclear components.

127. The answer is D. *(Wilson, ed 12. pp 1437–1443.)* Rheumatoid arthritis (RA) occurs in the fourth and fifth decades of life and affects women about three times as often as men. There is often a family history of RA. Insidious onset of inflammation affecting multiple joints, anorexia, fever, weight loss, and weakness occur in about two-thirds of patients; about one-third of patients will have disease in one or only a few joints. Where polyarticular disease occurs, it is usually found in a bilaterally symmetrical distribution and usually affects the metacarpophalangeal, wrist, elbow, knee, ankle, and metatarsophalangeal joints. The proximal interphalangeal joints are also often affected, but the distal interphalangeal joints are not; inflammation at the latter location suggests another disease, e.g., psoriatic arthritis. Patients with high-titer rheumatoid factor are predisposed to developing extraarticular manifestations of *rheumatoid disease* (this term, preferable to *rheumatoid arthritis*, accents the multisystem nature of the disease), such as rheumatoid nodules, which often occur near the olecranon bursa. Other extraarticular manifestations include nodular and fibrotic lung disease, scleritis, and vasculitis. Wasting of dorsal interosseous muscle is common when the metacarpophalangeal joints are inflamed; atrophy often occurs in muscles near inflamed joints, e.g., the quadriceps muscle.

128. The answer is B. *(Wilson, ed 12. pp 1443–1448.)* Scleroderma, or progressive systemic sclerosis, is a disease in which many organs may be damaged by the relentless deposition of fibrous connective tissue. Most frequently affected are the skin and blood vessels, but the gastrointestinal tract, lungs, kidneys, and heart are also commonly involved. Although scleroderma that is localized to the skin may be compatible with a normal life span, systemic involvement is often fatal. Gradual thickening of the skin is associated with loss of mobility that will eventually make it difficult to flex the finger joints normally. In addition and classically, telangiectasias are prominent. When muscles are involved in the sclerodermatous destructive process they are usually proximal muscle groups in a polymyositis-like syndrome. There has been much recent interest in the lung disease that commonly complicates the course of scleroderma. Pulmonary hypertension is common and may lead to cor pulmonale when pulmonary blood vessels are affected by the fibrotic process. However, interstitial pulmonary fibrosis can develop with alveolar involvement. Although this may represent the direct effects of the disease process, esophageal reflux is so common that a number of studies have demonstrated fibrotic changes in the lung secondary to the aspiration of gastric contents, particularly while the patient sleeps at night. In such cases surgical intervention may be necessary to protect the lungs. As fibrosis destroys the autonomic nerve supply to the intestinal tract, hypomotility and dilatation of the intestinal tract occur. Slowing the passage of food content through the intestinal tract may lead to a malabsorption syndrome. Obstruction due to intestinal fibrosis may occur. The CREST syndrome involves the deposition of calcium in the skin, the presence of Raynaud's phenomenon, esophageal hypomotility, sclerodactyly, and telangiectasis. It is of interest that while extensive myocardial dysfunction can occur secondary to fibrotic changes in the heart, this is extremely unusual in the CREST syndrome. Serologic evidence would suggest a different immunologic mechanism may be responsible for the CREST syndrome. Three forms of antinuclear antibody appear to be specific for scleroderma. Antibody to Scl-70 antigen as well as to the nuclear centromere and nucleolar antigens has been demonstrated. The anticentromere antibody is primarily seen in patients with the CREST form of the disease. Treatment of the disease is mainly symptomatic. Steroids do not help, but the malabsorption syndrome is frequently helped by the use of broad-spectrum antibiotics. Captopril, the oral angiotensin-converting enzyme inhibitor, has helped a number of patients with serious hypertension, and in severe ischemic crises sympathectomy has reversed some of the effects of the Raynaud's phenomenon.

129. The answer is C (2, 4). *(Wilson, ed 12. pp 1453-1455, 1482-1484.)* Five percent of patients suffering from psoriasis develop an arthritic syndrome. Usually the psoriasis is present for many years before joint inflammation develops, but occasionally arthritis may occur before the skin disease. The different syndromes associated with psoriatic arthritis are subgrouped according to the joints involved. At least 70 percent of patients with psoriatic arthritis have a monarticular or asymmetrical oligoarticular arthritis. The smaller joints in the hands and feet can be involved and a classic finding is the sausage-shaped digits produced when the flexor tendon sheaths in the fingers become swollen and inflamed. Fifteen percent of patients with psoriatic arthritis present with a seronegative rheumatoid arthritis-type picture. A third group of patients suffer from arthritis that is limited to the distal interphalangeal joints, and with this form pitting of the fingernails is characteristic. A rare form of psoriatic arthritis is associated with a destructive arthropathy. This form tends to occur in men more than women, although psoriatic arthritis in general is more common in females. Sacroiliitis and spondylitis also occur in association with psoriasis. There is a linkage with HLA-B27 but not as strongly as is seen in ankylosing spondylitis (65 percent in psoriatic disease, up to 95 percent in ankylosing spondylitis). Between 10 and 20 percent of patients with psoriatic arthritis have hyperuricemia, but this rarely leads to crystal formation in joints and is more a reflection of the severity of the skin disease. The treatment of this form of arthritis is similar to that of rheumatoid arthritis.

130. The answer is A (1, 2, 3). *(Wilson, ed 12. pp 101, 122–123, 1488–1489.)* All that hurts in and near a joint is not arthritis; another cause of pain may be inflammation of periarticular structures, like the bursa or tendons. Preceding inflammatory joint disease may predispose to tendinitis, especially if previous damage or splinting of the joint causes changes in the biomechanics of the shoulder apparatus. The rotator cuff consists of the supraspinatus, infraspinatus, teres minor, and subscapularis muscles (SITS). The supraspinatus is a long, thin muscle, whose central portion is poorly vascularized and often compressed by the underlying humeral head—a prime target for local damage and inflammation. Rotator cuff tendinitis may lead to "frozen shoulder." Most such patients will improve spontaneously within about 2 years. Hydroxyapatite crystals in the glenohumeral joint or in the tendons may occur and cause inflammation, with ultimate rotator cuff rupture or shoulder osteoarthritis. This is called the "Milwaukee shoulder syndrome," named after the city where it was first described.

131. The answer is A (1, 2, 3). *(Wilson, ed 12. pp 547, 655, 1485–1486, 1754, 2086.)* Charcot's joints occur in those conditions that are characterized by abnormalities of proprioception and deep pain sensation. A single joint is involved initially and other joints follow, the distribution being determined by the underlying neurologic disorder. In tabes dorsalis, the knees, hips, ankles, and lumbar spine are involved; in diabetes, the tarsometatarsal, metatarsophalangeal, and tarsal joints are affected; and in syringomyelia, the shoulders, elbows, and cervical spine reveal pathologic changes. The involved joints suffer recurrent fractures with secondary overgrowth of bone. Effusions, pain, and joint instability are the end results. Ultimately there may be total joint destruction with no residual joint structure remaining. Braces and treatment of the underlying disorder are the only effective therapies.

132. The answer is E (all). *(Wilson, ed 12. pp 1475–1479.)* The term *degenerative joint disease* is to be eschewed and replaced by the more proper *osteoarthritis*. The major characteristics of osteoarthritis are loss of joint cartilage and hypertrophy of bone, including subchondral sclerosis and osteophyte formation. Within osteoarthritic cartilage, there is a marked increase in metabolic activity owing to the increased rate of destruction of cartilage accompanied by an increased synthesis of cartilage matrix. The increased proteolytic activity in the joint space is associated with higher-than-normal levels of proteases, particularly cathepsin D and similar hydrolases. As the disease progresses, cartilage is steadily lost from the joint because anabolic processes are unable to keep up with catabolism. Thus, there is evidence to suggest that osteoarthritis has active metabolic processes at work, rather than being merely the end result of "wear and tear." Chronic occupational trauma to joints—

such as that encountered by air-hammer workers—may result in osteoarthritis in joints that usually are not involved in this disease, such as the wrists, elbows, and shoulders. The excessive secretion of growth hormone in patients with acromegaly is thought to be responsible for the thickening of synovial tissues and the overgrowth of joint cartilage that characterize the articular changes seen early in this disease. This cartilage is abnormal and is unable to effectively bear weight. If acromegaly is untreated, marked changes will occur in joints. Because routine laboratory tests cannot detect the abnormalities, radiologic observation of changes occurring in joints still provides the most useful information for arriving at a diagnosis of osteoarthritis.

133. The answer is E (all). *(Wilson, ed 12. pp 1449–1450.)* Sjögren's syndrome consists of the triad of keratoconjunctivitis sicca, xerostomia, and a connective tissue disorder. The diagnosis is proved by biopsy of a minor salivary gland, with demonstration of a lymphocytic infiltration plus glandular disruption. The connective tissue disease most commonly associated with the sicca complex is rheumatoid arthritis, but other diseases such as systemic lupus erythematosus, scleroderma, polymyositis, chronic active hepatitis, Waldenström's macroglobulinemia, pseudo-lymphoma, and malignant lymphoma may also be a part of this complex.

134. The answer is C (2, 4). *(Wilson, ed 12. pp 90–92, 1451–1453, 1483–1484.)* The HLA-B27 antigen is found on the leukocytes of 90 percent of patients with ankylosing spondylitis, but is also present in 7 percent of normal whites. Therefore, the routine use of this test in an individual is usually not valuable for diagnosing inflammatory joint disease. However, in population studies, 25 percent of those who are B27-positive will go on to experience clinical or roentgenographic evidence of spondylitis or sacroiliitis or both. B27 is also associated with psoriatic spondylitis, the spondylitis seen in inflammatory bowel disease, Reiter's syndrome, and anterior uveitis. The exact means by which B27 confers a risk of spondylitis is not known. Occasionally, anterior uveitis may be the first manifestation of ankylosing spondylitis. In the absence of any evidence of inflammation on x-ray or by erythrocyte sedimentation rate (ESR) or of any symptoms referrable to the gastrointestinal tract, an x-ray of the large bowel is not indicated. The diagnosis of ankylosing spondylitis cannot be made in this patient at this time, and, at any rate, gold has not been notable as an effective form of therapy in ankylosing spondylitis. Evidence of ankylosing spondylitis may develop over the course of time. No symptoms at this time suggest an inflammatory joint disease. No morning stiffness is noted and the pain occurs after strenuous exercise; if this were an inflammatory disease, morning stiffness and relief after exercise might be expected.

135. The answer is B (1, 3). *(Wilson, ed 12. pp 1475–1479.)* Osteoarthritis is the most common form of joint disease in adults. When all age groups are considered, men and women are equally affected. The pathologic process is characterized by fibrillation and flaking of articular cartilage and remodeling of subchondral bone to produce the characteristic picture of joint space narrowing, subchondral eburnation, and osteophyte formation. Joint trauma may initiate this disease even in young people. The joint fluid in osteoarthritis is noninflammatory in nature; it contains only a few hundred white cells with normal protein and glucose.

136. The answer is E (all). *(Wilson, ed 12. pp 325, 547–548, 667–669.)* Lyme disease was first recognized in 1975 when a clustering of cases of "juvenile rheumatoid arthritis" occurred around the southern Connecticut town of Lyme. Many of these patients had a distinctive skin rash, erythema chronicum migrans. This disease is of particular interest as it is the first arthritis known quite definitely to be triggered by an infectious agent that is associated in many patients with numerous extraarticular, severe, and chronic complications. In 1983 the organism responsible was identified as a spirochete later named *Borrelia burgdorferi*, which can be grown on Kelly's medium. Antibody responses to the organism may be delayed. Some patients with infectious mononucleosis, syphilis, yaws, other *Borrelia* infections, rheumatoid arthritis, and lupus have developed similar antibodies. The disease is not a new one, as similar cases had been described in Europe over 80 years ago. In recent times cases have been described in Europe and Australia. Lyme disease has been found in many states. Within states the distribution of Lyme disease is very uneven, with focal endemic areas. Although a lymphocytic meningoradiculitis has been found in Europe to be caused by direct invasion of a spirochete that seems identical to the one that causes Lyme arthritis, some of the complications of this disease may be autoimmune in nature. There are numerous immunologic abnormalities in patients with Lyme disease, which is therefore a particularly valuable model for studying the way an environmental agent can disturb immunoregulation. Cardiac conduction abnormalities occur in a small percentage of patients, but they can be severe, ranging from first-degree to complete heart block. The early neurologic complications consist most commonly of an aseptic meningitis but also encephalitis and cranial nerve disorders. A radiculoneuritis and myelitis have been observed. Months to many years after onset, dementia, encephalopathy, and neuropathy may occur. This is known as "tertiary neuroborreliosis" and is analogous to tertiary neurosyphilis and its latent phase. Tetracycline and penicillin are equally good as treatment of the early stages of the disease, but tetracycline appears to minimize the development of chronic complications involving the heart and nervous system.

137. The answer is D (4). *(Wilson, ed 12. pp 1271–1273, 1278, 1483–1484.)* The peripheral arthritis associated with inflammatory bowel disease is found in approximately 25 percent of cases, more commonly in Crohn's disease and especially when the regional enteritis involves the colon. The arthritis is nondeforming, monarticular or polyarticular, without definite symmetry, and migratory. The attacks may be acute and most frequently involve the knees and ankles, although any joint may be affected. Serologic tests are negative and synovial fluid findings are typical of an acute arthritis. Attacks usually parallel the disease activity of the colitis. Prognostically, complete resolution without deformities occurs within several weeks. This is in contrast to the spondylitis of inflammatory bowel disease, which may precede the colitis and whose activity is not related to the course of the underlying gastrointestinal dysfunction. The sacroiliitis and spondylitis of inflammatory bowel disease are much like that of ankylosing spondylitis on radiographic evaluation.

138-142. The answers are: 138-A, 139-C, 140-D, 141-B, 142-B. *(Wilson, ed 12. pp 314-317, 330, 375-379, 1144-1145, 1186, 1436-1437, 1441-1443, 1447, 1845, 1880.)* Drugs used in the treatment of rheumatoid arthritis are broadly classified as anti-inflammatory or remission-inducing (remittive) agents. Aspirin, a nonsteroidal anti-inflammatory agent that inhibits prostaglandin synthesis, is a commonly used first-line drug. The most frequent side effect is gastrointestinal distress.

Gold therapy is effective in many patients with rheumatoid arthritis, especially in those whose disease is of recent onset. Side effects, however, are significant and include a dermatitis that may lead to exfoliative dermatitis if treatment is not discontinued, stomatitis, the nephrotic syndrome, and bone marrow suppression. Patients' response to gold may be only temporary.

Low-dose prednisone may be very useful in controlling an acute flare of arthritis or in controlling the disease while waiting for a remittive agent to begin working. However, prednisone has significant toxicity, including osteoporosis.

The most significant side effect of chloroquine is deposition of the drug in the pigmented layer of the retina. Irreversible retinal degeneration may develop, and this has limited the use of this drug. Hydroxychloroquine (Plaquenil) is less frequently associated with retinopathy. Ophthalmic examinations are required every 6 months of therapy.

143-147. The answers are: 143-B, 144-D, 145-A, 146-C, 147-E. *(McCarty, ed 11. pp 1189-1196. Wilson, ed 12. pp 1040-1043, 1438-1445, 1457-1462.)* Wegener's granulomatosis is a granulomatous vasculitis of small arteries and veins that affects the lungs, sinuses, nasopharynx, and the kidneys, where it causes a focal and segmental glomerulonephritis. Other organs can also be damaged, including the skin, eyes, and nervous system. A recently described blood test, identifying antibodies to the cytoplasm of neutrophils, may prove to be of use in making the diagnosis. Treatment has been successful with steroids and cyclophosphamide. Recent evidence suggests that trimethoprim-sulfamethoxazole may also be effective, which raises the possibility that this drug combination may be killing a causative microorganism or may be modifying the immune response in some way.

Elderly people may have extensive atherosclerosis. Especially after an endovascular procedure (like vascular catheterization, grafting, or repair), some of the atheromatous material may embolize, usually to the skin, kidneys, and brain. This material is capable of fixing complement and thus causing vascular damage. The skin lesions—ecchymoses and necrosis—look much like vasculitis. Differentiation between cholesterol embolization and idiopathic vasculitis is important, since not only is the former not steroid-sensitive but there have been reports of increasing damage after the institution of steroid therapy.

Polyarteritis nodosa is a multisystem necrotizing vasculitis that, prior to the use of steroids and cyclophosphamide, was uniformly fatal. In 30 percent of patients, antecedent hepatitis B virus infection can be demonstrated; immune complexes containing the virus have been found in such patients and are likely pathogenetic.

Giant cell arteritis is a disease of elderly patients that classically affects the temporal arteries (thus, the old name, temporal arteritis). Giant cell arteritis, named for the presence of giant cells and granulomata disrupting the internal elastica of the vessel, may present with headache, anemia, a high ESR (although a normal ESR does *not* rule out the diagnosis), and occasionally a syndrome known as polymyalgia rheumatica. This includes stiffness, aching, and tenderness of the proximal muscles. These patients describe weakness of the hip and shoulder girdles, but there is no objective weakness of the muscles and the muscle enzymes are normal. Giant cell arteritis usually responds to steroid therapy, 45 to 60 mg per day of prednisone; polymyalgia rheumatica typically responds to low-dose prednisone, 10 to 15 mg per day.

First described in Japan and then in Turkey, Takayasu's arteritis is a granulomatous inflammation of the aorta and its main branches. Symptoms are due to local vascular occlusion; aortic regurgitation and systemic and pulmonary hypertension, as well as general symptoms of arthralgia, fatigue, malaise, anorexia, and weight loss, may occur. Surgery may be necessary to correct occlusive lesions.

148-152. The answers are: 148-C, 149-B, 150-A, 151-A, 152-B. *(Wilson, ed 12. pp 546, 1453-1455.)* Reiter's syndrome is characterized as a triad of seronegative, oligoarticular, asymmetric arthritis; conjunctivitis; and urethritis. The arthritis coupled with urethritis or cervicitis may be sufficient for the diagnosis. It is the most common cause of arthritis in young men. The syndrome develops in up to 3 percent of males with nongonococcal urethritis, in 2 to 3 percent of patients with bacillary dysentery, and in 20 percent of persons with the HLA-B27 antigen. While the pathogenesis is unclear, an infectious process of the urogenital tract (postvenereal Reiter's) or gut (postdysentery Reiter's) together with a particular genetic background may trigger the development of Reiter's syndrome.

The disorder usually begins with urethritis followed by conjunctivitis, which is usually minimal, and rheumatologic findings. The arthritis is usually acute, asymmetric, and oligoarticular and involves predominantly the joints of the lower extremities; tenosynovitis, dactylitis, and plantar fasciitis also occur. Painless, superficial oral mucosal and glans penile lesions occur in a third of patients; keratosis blennorrhagica occurs in up to 30 percent of postvenereal Reiter's syndrome patients but does not occur in postdysentery patients; circinate balanitis is a characteristic dermatitis of the glans penis.

The diagnosis of gonococcal arthritis is made if the organism is cultured from a mucosal site, typical pustular or hemorrhagic lesions are distributed primarily on the extremities, and a therapeutic antibiotic trial resolves the fevers and arthritis. The course is typically acute, typically involves joints of the upper extremities, and may be associated with uveitis. There is no linkage of HLA-B27 with this disease; thus, the frequency of HLA-B27 is the same as in the general population, 6 to 8 percent.

Pulmonary Disease

DIRECTIONS: Each question below contains five suggested responses. Select the **one best** response to each question.

153. A 64-year-old woman is found to have a left-sided pleural effusion on chest x-ray. Analysis of the pleural fluid reveals a ratio of concentration of total protein in pleural fluid to serum of 0.38, a lactic dehydrogenase (LDH) level of 125 IU, and a ratio of LDH concentration in pleural fluid to serum of 0.46. Which of the following disorders is most likely in this patient?

(A) Uremia
(B) Congestive heart failure
(C) Pulmonary embolism
(D) Sarcoidosis
(E) Systemic lupus erythematosus

154. A patient is found to have an unexpectedly high value for diffusing capacity. This finding is consistent with which of the following disorders?

(A) Anemia
(B) Cystic fibrosis
(C) Emphysema
(D) Intrapulmonary hemorrhage
(E) Pulmonary emboli

155. All the following statements concerning the pulmonary effects of radiation therapy are true EXCEPT

(A) symptoms of radiation pneumonitis usually become evident 2 to 3 months after the completion of radiation therapy
(B) frank hemoptysis is an uncommon symptom of radiation pneumonitis
(C) concomitant use of radiation and chemotherapy does not increase the risk of developing radiation pneumonitis
(D) the earliest radiologic change after irradiation of the thorax is a radiolucency of the irradiated area
(E) a second course of radiation therapy to the lung is more likely to precipitate acute radiation pneumonitis than the first

156. All the following are indicative of a *severe* asthmatic attack EXCEPT

(A) silent chest
(B) hypercapnia
(C) thoracoabdominal paradox (paradoxical respiration)
(D) pulsus paradoxus of 5 mmHg
(E) altered mental status

157. A 32-year-old black woman without a significant past medical history is referred for a dry cough of 3 weeks' duration. She is afebrile, and physical examination is entirely normal except for the presence of several palpable anterior cervical lymph nodes. A chest roentgenogram reveals significant bilateral hilar adenopathy and clear lung fields. A serum Ca^{2+} is 9.5 mg/dL and a purified protein derivative (PPD) test is nonreactive. A lymph node biopsy reveals granulomas and a stain for acid-fast bacilli (AFB) is negative. All the following statements regarding this patient's current medical condition are true EXCEPT

(A) the angiotensin converting enzyme (ACE) level is a good predictor of the severity of the illness and determines the overall prognosis
(B) approximately 70 percent of patients with this disorder will improve or remain stable without medical therapy
(C) pulmonary function tests in this patient are likely to be abnormal
(D) other organs that may become involved in the disease process in this patient include the skin, heart, liver, spleen, and eye
(E) the etiologic agent responsible for causing this patient's medical problem is not known

158. A 40-year-old man without a significant past medical history comes to the emergency room with a 3-day history of fever, shaking chills with a 15-min episode of rigor, nonproductive cough, and anorexia, as well as the development of right-sided pleuritic chest pain and shortness of breath over the last 12 h. A chest roentgenogram reveals a consolidated right middle lobe infiltrate and a CBC shows an elevated neutrophil count with many band forms present. Which of the following statements regarding pneumonia in this patient is correct?

(A) Sputum culture is more helpful than sputum Gram stain in choosing empiric antibiotic therapy
(B) If the Gram stain revealed numerous gram-positive diplococci, numerous white blood cells, and few epithelial cells, penicillin would be adequate empiric therapy
(C) Although *Streptococcus pneumoniae* is the agent most likely to be the cause of this patient's pneumonia, this diagnosis would be very unlikely if blood cultures were negative
(D) The absence of rigors would rule out a diagnosis of pneumococcal pneumonia
(E) The absence of clinical improvement after 72 h of penicillin therapy would rule out the diagnosis of pneumococcal pneumonia

159. The hallmark of asthma that distinguishes it from other obstructive airway diseases is that in asthma

(A) hyperinflation is present on chest roentgenogram
(B) airway obstruction is reversible
(C) hypoxia occurs as a consequence of ventilation-perfusion mismatch
(D) the FEV_1/FVC ratio is reduced
(E) exacerbation often occurs as a result of an upper respiratory tract infection

160. Factors known to exacerbate obstructive sleep apnea include all the following EXCEPT

(A) consumption of ethanol
(B) benzodiazepines taken orally at bedtime
(C) weight gain
(D) orally administered tricyclic antidepressants
(E) supine body position

161. A 32-year-old white woman is found to have a widened mediastinum on a routine chest roentgenogram. She is completely asymptomatic. A CT scan demonstrates that a mass is in the anterior mediastinum. The best approach to managing this patient would be to

(A) do nothing at this time since most anterior mediastinal masses are benign and she is presently asymptomatic
(B) refer the patient to an oncologist since most anterior mediastinal masses are malignant and not resectable at the time of presentation
(C) perform a Tensilon test since most anterior mediastinal tumors in this age group are thymomas associated with myasthenia gravis
(D) refer the patient to a thoracic surgeon for thoracotomy and removal of the mediastinal mass
(E) perform radiation therapy initially to shrink the tumor, then follow with thoracotomy

DIRECTIONS: Each question below contains four suggested responses of which **one or more** is correct. Select

A	if	**1, 2, and 3**	are correct
B	if	**1 and 3**	are correct
C	if	**2 and 4**	are correct
D	if	**4**	is correct
E	if	**1, 2, 3, and 4**	are correct

162. Correct statements concerning oxygen toxicity include which of the following?

(1) Breathing 100% oxygen may result in a large right-to-left shunt
(2) Changes in pulmonary function tests are not seen when lungs are exposed to less than 0.5 atmosphere of oxygen
(3) Changes in pulmonary function may become evident after 24 h of exposure at 1.0 atmosphere of oxygen
(4) The oxygen molecule is extremely toxic to the lung and is primarily responsible for the development of pulmonary fibrosis during breathing of 1.0 atmosphere of oxygen

163. True statements concerning theophylline include that

(1) at therapeutic concentrations, inhibition of phosphodiesterase activity is insignificant
(2) cimetidine causes a marked decrease in theophylline clearance
(3) it augments the ventilatory response to hypoxia
(4) patients with congestive heart failure will frequently require higher doses of theophylline to achieve the desired therapeutic effect

164. True statements concerning Wegener's granulomatosis include that

(1) hilar adenopathy is commonly the initial chest x-ray abnormality
(2) the disease is never limited solely to the respiratory tract
(3) disease involvement in organs other than the kidney and respiratory tract is a rare finding
(4) multiple, bilateral nodular infiltrates are typical

165. Lung abscesses are characterized by which of the following statements?

(1) They are most commonly caused by a single anaerobic bacterium
(2) They are most commonly caused by aspiration
(3) Surgical resection reduces the length of antibiotic therapy
(4) They are more commonly noted in the lower lobes, particularly the superior segments

SUMMARY OF DIRECTIONS

A	B	C	D	E
1, 2, 3 only	1, 3 only	2, 4 only	4 only	All are correct

166. True statements concerning complications of tracheostomies include which of the following?

(1) Airway colonization with *Pseudomonas* or gram-negative enteric organisms occurs in a large proportion of patients
(2) Tracheal stenosis occurs less frequently in tracheostomies compared with prolonged endotracheal intubation
(3) Symptoms of tracheal stenosis may develop years after extubation
(4) Pneumothorax will not occur because the tracheal incision is far from the pleura

167. A 28-year-old man enters the hospital with cough and fever. His admission x-ray is shown below. Acid-fast organisms, subsequently identified as *Mycobacterium tuberculosis*, are seen on a smear. Correct statements regarding the pathophysiology of this patient's infection include which of the following?

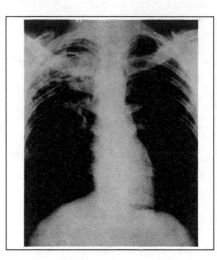

(1) The initial exposure probably occurred at a time remote from the current symptoms
(2) The location of the current process probably resulted from inspiration of aerosolized droplets into the upper lobe
(3) Necrosis of the pulmonary lesion with cavity formation is a common complication of his condition
(4) Although coughing is the most common way of spreading this infection, sneezing and even talking have been implicated in disease transmission

DIRECTIONS: Each group of questions below consists of lettered headings followed by a set of numbered items. For each numbered item select the **one** lettered heading with which it is **most** closely associated. Each lettered heading may be used **once, more than once, or not at all.**

Questions 168–172

For each clinical picture below, select the arterial blood gas and pH values with which it is most likely to be associated.

	pH	P_{O_2}	P_{CO_2}
(A)	7.54	75	28
(B)	7.15	78	92
(C)	7.06	36	95
(D)	7.06	108	13
(E)	7.39	48	54

168. A 30-year-old obese female bus driver develops sudden pleuritic left-sided chest pain and dyspnea

169. A 60-year-old heavy smoker has severe chronic bronchitis and peripheral edema and cyanosis

170. A 22-year-old drug-addicted man is brought to the emergency room by friends who were unable to awaken him

171. A 62-year-old man who has chronic bronchitis and chest pain is given oxygen via mask in the ambulance en route to the hospital and becomes lethargic in the emergency room

172. A 20-year-old man with diabetes mellitus comes to the emergency room with diffuse abdominal pain, tachypnea, and a fever of 104°F (40°C)

Questions 173–177

For each set of findings below, select the disease with which it is most likely to be associated.

    (A) Asthma
    (B) Rheumatoid arthritis
    (C) α_1-Antitrypsin deficiency
    (D) Cystic fibrosis
    (E) Sarcoidosis

173. Low levels of glucose in pleural effusions

174. Bronchiectasis and severe hemoptysis as frequent complications of clinical course

175. Presence of the mucoid strain of *Pseudomonas aeruginosa*

176. Development of severe liver disease that is usually associated with, but may be independent of, lung disease

177. Development of symptoms after ingestion of tartrazine yellow or aspirin

DIRECTIONS: The group of questions below consists of four lettered headings followed by a set of numbered items. For each numbered item select

A	if the item is associated with	(A) **only**
B	if the item is associated with	(B) **only**
C	if the item is associated with	**both** (A) and (B)
D	if the item is associated with	**neither** (A) nor (B)

Each lettered heading may be used **once, more than once, or not at all.**

Questions 178–181

(A) Rheumatoid arthritis
(B) Scleroderma
(C) Both
(D) Neither

178. Acute pneumonia

179. Diffuse interstitial fibrosis

180. Pleural effusion

181. Pulmonary nodules

Pulmonary Disease

Answers

153. The answer is B. *(Fishman, ed 2. p 2134.)* Classifying a pleural effusion as either a transudate or an exudate is useful in identifying the underlying disorder. Pleural fluid is exudative if it has any one of the following three properties: a ratio of concentration of total protein in pleural fluid to serum greater than 0.5, an absolute value of LDH greater than 200 IU, or a ratio of LDH concentration in pleural fluid to serum greater than 0.6. Causes of exudative effusions include malignancy, pulmonary embolism, pneumonia, tuberculosis, abdominal disease, collagen vascular diseases, uremia, Dressler's syndrome, and chylothorax. Exudative effusions may also be drug-induced. If none of the aforementioned properties are met, the effusion is a transudate. Differential diagnosis includes congestive heart failure, nephrotic syndrome, cirrhosis, Meigs's syndrome, and hydronephrosis. It is important to note that congestive heart failure, pneumonia, malignancy, and pulmonary embolic disease account for more than 90 percent of all pleural effusions.

154. The answer is D. *(Fishman, ed 2. p 2497.)* The diffusing capacity provides an estimate of the rate at which carbon monoxide moves by diffusion from alveolar gas to combine with hemoglobin in the red blood cells. It is interpreted as an index of the surface area engaged in alveolar-capillary diffusion. Measurement of diffusing capacity of the lung (DL_{CO}) is done by having the person inspire a low concentration of carbon monoxide. The rate of uptake of the gas by the blood is calculated from the difference between the inspired and expired concentrations. The test can be performed during a single 10-s breath-holding or during a minute of steady-state breathing. The diffusing capacity is defined as the amount of carbon monoxide transferred per minute per millimeter of mercury of driving pressure. Normal values hover about 20 mL/min per mmHg at rest and 60 mL/min per mmHg on exercise. Primary parenchymal disorders and removal of lung tissue decrease the diffusing surface area and cause the DL_{CO} to be low. Conversely, polycythemia and intrapulmonary hemorrhage tend to increase the value for diffusing capacity.

155. The answer is C. *(Gross, Ann Intern Med 86:81–92, 1977.)* Radiation administered to the thorax in the treatment of patients with breast cancer, lung cancer, Hodgkin's disease, or lymphoma may result in adverse effects on lung and pleura. The incidence and severity of damage are related to two major factors: the greater the volume of lung irradiated, the greater the likelihood of clinical disturbance; and the amount of damage produced is more a function of the rate at which the total dose is delivered than of the total dose, as increasing fractionation allows repair of sublethal damage. The clinical syndrome is divided into two phases: radiation pneumonitis, which occurs 2 to 6 months after radiation therapy, and radiation fibrosis, which follows it and is usually established by 12 months. Symptoms of radiation pneumonitis begin insidiously and usually consist of a harsh cough and dyspnea; frank hemoptysis is uncommon. Nearly all patients with radiation pneumonitis will develop radiation fibrosis and in most cases this will be asymptomatic. However, in severe cases, dyspnea, orthopnea, cyanosis, and clubbing may occur. Concomitant chemotherapy, repeat courses of radiation, and steroid withdrawal all may potentiate the damaging effects of radiation.

156. The answer is D. *(Murray, pp 1047–1050.)* It is extremely important to accurately determine the severity of an exacerbation of asthma since the major cause of death from asthma is the underestimation of the severity of a particular episode either by the patient or the physician. Silent chest is a particularly ominous finding because the airway constriction is so great that airflow is insufficient to generate wheezing. Hypercapnia and thoracoabdominal paradox almost always are indicative of exhaustion and respiratory muscle failure or fatigue and generally need to be aggressively treated with mechanical ventilation. Altered mental status is frequently seen with severe hypoxia or hypercapnia, and ventilatory support is usually required. An increased pulsus paradoxus may also be a sign of severe asthma, as it increases with greater respiratory effort and generation of more negative intrathoracic pressures during inspiration. However, a pulsus paradoxus of up to 8 to 10 mmHg is considered normal; thus, a value of 5 mmHg would not be indicative of a severe episode of asthma.

157. The answer is A. *(Murray, pp 1486–1497.)* The patient has a history, physical examination, chest roentgenogram, and lymph node biopsy consistent with sarcoidosis. No etiologic agent responsible for causing sarcoidosis has been identified, although it has been suggested that transmissible, airborne substances and genetic factors may be involved. The hallmark of the disease is a granuloma with inflammatory regions that may occur in any area of the body. This leads to a varied presentation in this disorder. Most typically, sarcoidosis presents as an abnormal chest roentgenogram with hilar and paratracheal lymphadenopathy. The lung fields may be clear or demonstrate parenchymal disease. Occasionally, patients may present without lymphadenopathy and with parenchymal disease alone ("burned-out" sarcoidosis). Despite the significant abnormalities on chest roentgenogram, physical examination of the lungs is generally normal, and the major abnormality on examination, if present, is lymphadenopathy. In symptomatic patients, the affected organ or organs dictate the presentation of the disease. Since pulmonary involvement is most common, dry cough and mild dyspnea are the symptoms most often noted, although nonspecific constitutional symptoms, such as weight loss, fatigue, and anorexia are occasionally seen. Other organ systems involved in sarcoidosis include the skin, eye, heart, nervous system, gastrointestinal tract, and kidney.

Diagnosis of sarcoidosis is generally accomplished with tissue biopsy confirming granuloma and without evidence of tuberculosis or other infectious granulomatous diseases. Transbronchial biopsy of the lung during fiberoptic bronchoscopy is an excellent way of making the diagnosis, as a positive result will be obtained in 85 to 90 percent of patients with parenchymal radiographic abnormalities and in 50 to 60 percent of patients with hilar adenopathy alone. Lymph node biopsy may also provide an excellent and reasonably noninvasive way of establishing the diagnosis, although a number of false positive results have been reported. An accurate, but more invasive method of making the diagnosis is mediastinoscopy. The use of angiotensin converting enzyme (ACE) in establishing the diagnosis and in determining prognosis has not proved reliable since there is a wide variation in ACE levels in patients and elevations of ACE have been noted in various other illnesses. However, following the ACE level in an individual patient may occasionally be helpful in determining response to medical treatment.

Approximately 70 percent of patients with sarcoidosis either spontaneously remit or have a stable disease course over an extended period of time. Only about 30 percent show progression of symptoms, usually over a period of 5 to 10 years, although some patients may have a rapid downhill course with death due to respiratory failure in several months. Therefore, only a minority of patients need to be medically treated, usually with high-dose oral steroids. Patients are usually treated only if they are symptomatic (uncontrolled cough, anorexia), have hypercalcemia, have involvement in organ systems in which granulomata may lead to dangerous sequelae (heart, liver, and eye), or have evidence of worsening pulmonary status. Pulmonary function studies are frequently abnormal in these patients, even when they are minimally symptomatic, with the carbon monoxide–diffusing capacity most often abnormal. In more severely affected patients, there is evidence of pulmonary restriction with a decrease in lung volumes, and serial lung volumes and diffusing capacity may aid in determining optimal steroid dose and length of therapy.

158. The answer is B. *(Murray, pp 811–814.)* Pneumonia is a common disorder and is a major cause of death, particularly in hospitalized, elderly patients. Before choosing empiric therapy for presumed pneumonia, it is necessary to know the age of the patient, whether the infection is community-acquired or nosocomial, and whether there are any underlying debilitating illnesses. Community-acquired pneumonias in patients over the age of 35 are most likely due to *Streptococcus pneumoniae*, *Legionella* species (e.g., *pneumophila*), and *Haemophilus influenzae*. In the case outlined, the history is strongly consistent with pneumococcal pneumonia, manifest by a short prodrome, shaking chills with rigor, fever, chest pain, sparse sputum production associated with cough, and a consolidated lobar infiltrate on chest roentgenogram. The most reliable method of making an early diagnosis of pneumococcal pneumonia is seeing gram-positive diplococci on an adequate sputum (many white cells, few epithelial cells). Sputum culture is often not reliable in this disorder, since the organism may be easily overgrown. Blood cultures are positive in only about 20 percent of patients, and when positive, may be indicative of a more severe case. Although rigors are common and may be indicative of pneumococcal bacteremia, the absence of rigors does not rule out the diagnosis. Intravenous penicillin is usually the treatment of choice, and the classic response is rapid clinical improvement, frequently within 24 to 48 h. However, it has been appreciated with greater frequency that many patients, particularly older or debilitated patients, may not show clinical improvement for up to 7 days after beginning appropriate antibiotic therapy.

159. The answer is B. *(Murray, pp 1032–1068.)* Asthma is an incompletely understood inflammatory process involving the lower airways and resulting in bronchoconstriction and excess production of mucus, which lead to increased airway resistance and occasionally respiratory failure and death. During acute exacerbations of asthma and in other obstructive lung diseases, such as chronic obstructive pulmonary disease, hyperinflation may be present on chest roentgenogram, hypoxia is common and usually a result of ventilation-perfusion mismatch, the FEV_1/FVC is reduced, and exacerbations are frequently precipitated by upper airway infections. Only in asthma is the airway obstruction completely reversible.

160. The answer is D. *(Murray, pp 1845–1850.)* Obstructive sleep apnea (OSA) is a disease of abnormal respiratory control that has only been recognized for about 15 years. It is a very common disorder and may affect as many as 5 percent of the adult male population between the ages of 40 and 65. The typical presentation is an obese, middle-aged man with a short neck, a history of heavy snoring and excessive daytime sleepiness (hypersomnolence), and occasionally evidence of right heart failure. The etiology of OSA is not entirely known but is felt to involve a relative relaxation of upper airway dilator muscles during sleep, which leads to pharyngeal airway collapse during inspiration, when there is a negative intraluminal upper airway pressure. When the airway collapses there is no airflow (apnea); this leads to hypercapnia and hypoxia, which cause constant arousals from sleep (sleep fragmentation), inadequate deep sleep and rapid-eye-movement (REM) sleep time, and thus hypersomnolence. Until recently, there were few treatment options, with bypass of the upper airway by tracheostomy reserved for severe cases. Tricyclic antidepressants have been tried with limited success and probably work by reducing REM sleep time, a period of sleep in which obstructive apneic events are common. The most promising results have come from the recent use of nasal continuous positive airway pressure (nasal CPAP), which acts as a pneumatic splint to prevent pharyngeal airway collapse. Approximately 80 percent of patients with OSA respond to this treatment; however, many patients become noncompliant with nasal CPAP as their symptoms begin to dissipate. Uvulopalatopharyngoplasty (UPPP) is a procedure in which excess upper airway tissue is surgically removed in an attempt to increase the baseline size of the pharynx. The short-term results have been somewhat disappointing, with a success rate of about 50 percent and significant postoperative morbidity. Dental appliances have not had consistent results in treating OSA and are not usually employed in the initial treatment plan. Perhaps the best and often overlooked treatment strategy is weight loss, which may end the obstructive episodes entirely in certain subjects. Treatment is also aimed at avoidance of exacerbating factors of OSA. Ethanol and benzodiazepines both relax the genioglossus (tongue) muscle, a major pharyngeal dilator, and worsen OSA. In addition, supine body position seems to exacerbate sleep apnea by passively allowing the tongue to fall backwards secondary to gravity, making the pharyngeal airway smaller and more likely to obstruct.

161. The answer is D. *(Murray, pp 1819–1829.)* The mediastinum represents the space between the two pleural cavities and contains numerous structures from different organ systems. Therefore, there is a wide range of mediastinal pathology. When considering mediastinal masses, as in the case illustrated, the most useful method of characterizing the potential pathology is to divide the mediastinum into anterior, middle, and posterior and then localize the mass into one of these compartments. Both malignant and benign neoplasms arise in each segment of the mediastinum, but tumor type and frequency of malignancy are dependent upon both the location of the tumor in the mediastinum and the age of the patient. Tumors arising in the anterior mediastinum, the region most common for malignancy, include thymomas, germ-cell tumors, lymphomas, thyroid and parathyroid tumors, and mesenchymal tumors. It should be noted that with the exception of lymphomas, these tumors may be malignant or benign. Thymomas are the most common anterior mediastinal mass, and the association with myasthenia is reported to be between 10 and 50 percent. Therefore, patients with anterior mediastinal masses and symptoms consistent with myasthenia gravis should have appropriate testing to establish the diagnosis. Lesions arising in the middle mediastinum are usually benign and consist of developmental cysts, vascular enlargements, and diaphragmatic hernias, although enlarged lymph nodes from both benign and malignant processes can occur. In the posterior mediastinum, almost all lesions arise from neural tissue and are classified according to the specific tissue of origin. Most of these lesions are benign in adults, but up to 50 percent of these neoplasms may be malignant in children. Benign lesions may produce symptoms, including chest pain from nerve or bone erosion, dyspnea from tracheal compression, and neurologic deficits secondary to spinal cord compression.

Since mediastinal masses may be malignant or benign, and since even benign lesions may have significant symptoms, the goal of therapy has in general been surgical removal. In certain cases, closed chest biopsy may be appropriate as a diagnostic tool (tuberculosis, sarcoidosis) and may obviate the need for thoracotomy.

The outcome from mediastinal masses is generally favorable, since a majority of these lesions are benign. However, the results for many of the malignant neoplasms are also good, especially if the tumor is well encapsulated at the time of thoracotomy. Preoperative radiation or chemotherapy is not usually performed for most mediastinal masses.

162.   The answer is A (1, 2, 3). *(Fishman, ed 2. pp 2331-2337.)* Pulmonary oxygen toxicity is related to both the tension of administered oxygen and the duration of exposure. While human trials are not possible, indirect analyses have led to several conclusions: Oxygen toxicity does not usually occur in patients exposed to less than 0.5 atmosphere, and an FI_{O_2} of 1.0 should be given for the shortest possible duration. Furthermore, an FI_{O_2} of 1.0 may actually decrease arterial O_2 content by causing absorption atelectasis in those regions of the lung with low V/Q ratios. With time, exposure to a high FI_{O_2} causes a tracheobronchitis that progresses within a few days to pulmonary interstitial edema (noncardiogenic pulmonary edema) and finally to pulmonary fibrosis. Oxygen toxicity is not caused directly by the oxygen molecule, which is relatively nonreactive. It is generally felt to be caused by toxic free radicals of oxygen, produced from complete reduction of molecular oxygen.

163.   The answer is A (1, 2, 3). *(Fishman, ed 2. p 1314.)* Theophylline, a methylxanthine, is a frequently used drug in airway obstruction. One of its effects is to inhibit phosphodiesterase activity; however, at therapeutic concentrations, this inhibition is minimal and inadequate to explain the bronchodilation seen. Thus the mechanism responsible for bronchodilation from theophylline is unknown. Other effects of theophylline include improvement of diaphragmatic contractility and augmentation of the ventilatory response to hypoxia. Theophylline metabolism is altered by many drugs. Cimetidine, erythromycin, and birth control pills all reduce its clearance, while phenobarbital and phenytoin increase its clearance. In addition, theophylline dosage must be reduced in liver disease and congestive heart failure and must be increased in cigarette smokers and children.

164.   The answer is D (4). *(Fishman, ed 2. pp 1128-1136.)* Wegener's granulomatosis is characterized by glomerulonephritis together with a granulomatous vasculitis of the upper and lower respiratory tracts. Many other organ systems may typically be involved, including eyes, ears, skin, heart, and nervous system. Patients typically present with an upper airway illness related to persistent rhinorrhea and bilateral pulmonary infiltrates. Rarely is there functional renal impairment on presentation. Lung biopsy reveals the presence of granulomata and vasculitis, although, rarely, either may exist alone. The characteristic lung findings are multiple, bilateral nodular infiltrates that tend to cavitate. Twenty percent of patients have pleural effusions. Pulmonary calcifications are rare and hilar adenopathy is not a feature. On pulmonary function testing, airflow obstruction, reduced lung volumes, and an abnormal diffusing capacity are common findings. Without therapy, mortality is 90 percent in 2 years. A variant of systemic Wegener's granulomatosis, called *limited Wegener's*, has disease involvement limited to the respiratory tract. This variant may have a better overall prognosis than the systemic variety. Treatment for systemic

Wegener's granulomatosis is with prednisone, frequently with the addition of cyclophosphamide or azathioprine, especially if there is evidence of renal involvement. In limited Wegener's granulomatosis, there are several records of arrest of the disease process with trimethoprim-sulfamethoxazole treatment alone.

165. The answer is C (2, 4). *(Fishman, ed 2. pp 1505–1515.)* Lung abscess is characterized by destruction of lung parenchyma secondary to a suppurative inflammatory process resulting in cavitary lesions. Frequent predisposing factors include aspiration, periodontal disease, bronchiectasis, bacteremia, and intra-abdominal infection. Anaerobic abscesses, which are most common and are usually caused by more than one organism, typically have an indolent course, while those caused by *Staphylococcus aureus, Streptococcus pyogenes,* or *Klebsiella* have a more sudden presentation. Lung abscesses secondary to another process such as bacterial endocarditis or subphrenic infection may be dominated by the clinical presentation of the underlying pathology. Approximately one-third of lung abscesses are complicated by empyema. Treatment involves 2 to 4 months of antimicrobial therapy for complete resolution; surgical resection is contraindicated early in the disease process. A new treatment modality, currently under investigation, is percutaneous drainage of the abscess under radiologic guidance.

166. The answer is B (1, 3). *(Heffner, Chest 90:269–273, 430–435, 1986.)* Tracheostomy is one of the more frequent surgical procedures; indications include upper airway obstruction and long-term mechanical ventilation. While mortality is low, a number of complications are recognized. Because pleural extension into the neck may occur, especially in patients with emphysema, pneumothorax is not uncommon and develops in up to 5 percent of patients. Tracheal stenoses result from excessive cuff pressures and form as the tracheal injury heals. However, since both endotracheal and tracheostomy tubes use low-pressure cuffs, the risk of stenosis is equal. They manifest as dyspnea on exertion, cough, difficulty in clearing secretions, and stridor and may present several months to several years after extubation. Various forms of bleeding and tracheoesophageal fistulas are other noted complications.

167. The answer is B (1, 3). *(Fishman, ed 2. pp 1821–1840.)* The patient described in the question has active tuberculosis. The causative organism is initially inhaled by droplet aerosol into the lower lobes. A primary, usually asymptomatic infection ensues. Organisms are spread subsequently by hematogenous or lymphatic dissemination or both to other foci and grow best in those areas with a high oxygen tension, such as the upper lobe. Necrosis is part of the characteristic tissue reaction to infection. Symptomatic disease may then occur at these distant locations later in life. As the organism spreads by droplet aerosol, isolation of the patient becomes mandatory, preferably in a room with ultraviolet radiation. Coughing is usually the most effective method of spreading infection, as droplet nuclei of a size that can be inhaled are generated. Sneezing and talking usually produce droplet nuclei too large to reach the alveoli, where they are infectious.

168–172.   The answers are: 168-A, 169-E, 170-C, 171-B, 172-D. *(Murray, pp 211–230.)* The blood gas values associated with pulmonary embolism may vary tremendously. The most consistent finding is acute respiratory alkalosis. It is important to note that hypoxemia, although frequently found, need not be present.

In severe chronic lung disease, the presence of hypercapnia leads to a compensatory increase in serum bicarbonate. Thus, significant hypercapnia may be present with an arterial pH close to normal, but will never be *completely* corrected.

Acute respiratory acidosis may occur secondary to respiratory depression after drug overdose. Hypoventilation is associated with hypoxia, hypercapnia, and severe, uncompensated acidosis.

In the presence of long-standing lung disease, respiration may become regulated by hypoxia rather than by altered carbon dioxide tension and arterial pH, as in normal people. Thus, the unmonitored administration of oxygen may lead to respiratory suppression, as in the patient described in the question, resulting in acute and chronic respiratory acidosis.

Young patients with type I diabetes mellitus may present with rapid onset of diabetic ketoacidosis (DKA), usually secondary to a systemic infection. These patients usually are maximally ventilating, as indicated by a very low arterial P_{CO_2}; however, they remain acidotic secondary to the severe metabolic ketoacidosis associated with this process. In general, these patients are not hypoxic unless the underlying infection is pneumonia.

173–177.   The answers are: 173-B, 174-D, 175-D, 176-C, 177-A. *(Wilson, ed 12. pp 1047–1053, 1072–1076, 1343, 1437–1443, 1463–1469.)* Asthma is predominantly an inflammatory lower airway process. Frequent triggers of airway inflammation and thus asthma include infection, inhaled allergens, and processes that cool or dry the airways, such as exercise and exposure to cold weather. In addition, certain chemicals, such as aspirin (but not sodium or magnesium salicylate) and tartrazine yellow, have been implicated in the development of bronchospasm in certain patients.

Pleural effusions are not unusual in patients with rheumatoid arthritis. A history of pleurodynia that would suggest an antecedent inflammatory pleuritis is not always obtained, but characteristically the pleural fluid, which is sterile, will contain a high level of lactic dehydrogenase and a low glucose concentration. Other pulmonary phenomena associated with rheumatoid arthritis include diffuse interstitial fibrosis and the occurrence of individual or clustered nodules in the lung parenchyma.

The fatality rate for patients with cystic fibrosis is lower today than in previous years; currently, the average life span of patients afflicted with this disease is 19 years. Chronic lung infections, however, are almost universal. The most common and difficult to treat of such infections is caused by the mucoid strain of *Pseudomonas aeruginosa*. It is doubtful whether any form of antibiotic combination is effective in such patients. Distressing and chronic coughing is one of the major problems of patients with cystic fibrosis. Liver disease, particularly biliary cirrhosis, may develop in these patients. Common pulmonary complications include bronchiectasis, severe hemoptysis, and allergic bronchopulmonary aspergillosis.

The incidence of liver disease associated with a deficiency of α_1-antitrypsin is much higher than with *Pseudomonas aeruginosa* infections. Patients with liver disease secondary to α_1-antitrypsin deficiency usually, but not always, have accompanying panacinar emphysema.

Sarcoidosis is a nonspecific granulomatous disease of unknown etiology. Blacks and Mediterranean peoples appear to be predisposed. The most commonly involved organs—after the lungs— are liver, eye, spleen, skin, and kidney. The most characteristic presentation is a patient with a nonproductive cough with bilateral hilar adenopathy on chest x-ray. Treatment with prednisone is usually reserved for patients with diminishing pulmonary function, evidenced by reduced diffusing capacity or reduced lung volumes; 70 to 80 percent of untreated, stable patients will spontaneously remit.

178-181. The answers are: 178-D, 179-C, 180-A, 181-A. *(Fishman, ed 2. pp 645-656.)* Rheumatoid arthritis is a chronic inflammatory disease characterized by a symmetric polyarthritis affecting the small joints of the hands and feet as well as the large peripheral joints. Systemic features include fever, malaise, weight loss, and easy fatigability. Laboratory abnormalities include a normocytic, hypochromic anemia, diffuse hypergammaglobulinemia, hypoalbuminemia, and an elevated erythrocyte sedimentation rate. The pulmonary manifestations recognized to be part of the syndrome of rheumatoid arthritis are pleurisy with or without effusion, intrapulmonary rheumatoid nodules, rheumatoid pneumoconiosis, diffuse interstitial fibrosis, and bronchiolitis; ventilatory insufficiency is rare.

Scleroderma is a systemic, often progressive disorder of connective tissue. Presenting manifestations usually include Raynaud's phenomenon, thickening of the skin of the fingers, or musculoskeletal symptoms. The visceral organs affected include the gastrointestinal tract, kidneys, heart, and lungs. Pulmonary manifestations are pleural thickening, diffuse interstitial fibrosis, primary pulmonary vasculopathy, and ventilatory insufficiency. The diffusing capacity and the lung volumes are frequently decreased; respiratory failure is an occasional and important consequence of pulmonary disease in scleroderma.

Cardiology

DIRECTIONS: Each question below contains five suggested responses. Select the **one best** response to each question.

182. Hypertension is widely regarded as a major risk factor in the development of coronary heart disease. All the following statements regarding the association of hypertension and coronary heart disease are correct EXCEPT

(A) patients with mild hypertension account for approximately 60 percent of the premature deaths attributable to this risk factor

(B) a 10-mmHg rise in mean arterial pressure results in approximately a 30 percent rise in risk of coronary heart disease

(C) for all age groups and races in both sexes, a graded, incremental risk of fatal or nonfatal myocardial infarction has been demonstrated at diastolic blood pressures below the conventional 90-mmHg cutoff

(D) hypertension medications may have unfavorable effects on other coronary heart disease risk factors such as blood lipids and glucose and on cardiac rhythm disturbances

(E) the pharmacotherapeutic treatment of diastolic hypertension in the range of 90 to 105 mmHg has been shown to favorably influence morbidity and mortality of coronary heart disease

183. All the following statements regarding hypersensitive carotid sinus syndrome are correct EXCEPT

(A) ventricular asystole lasting 3 s or longer during carotid sinus stimulation characterizes cardioinhibitory carotid sinus hypersensitivity

(B) a drop in systolic blood pressure equal to or greater than 50 mmHg, or greater than 30 mmHg in association with reproducible symptoms, characterizes vasodepressor carotid sinus hypersensitivity

(C) intrinsic sinus nodal dysfunction is generally recognized as the major culprit in asystole in the hypersensitive carotid sinus syndrome

(D) mixed vasodepressor and cardioinhibitory carotid sinus hypersensitivity may account for recurrent episodes of syncope following pacemaker implantation for ventricular asystole in this syndrome

(E) pharmacotherapeutic agents such as beta-adrenergic blocking drugs, digitalis glycosides, α-methyldopa, and clonidine may accentuate cardioinhibitory and vasodepressor responses

184. A 25-year-old woman is seen by her physician because of progressive dyspnea, fatigue, and syncope on exertion. She has no history of rheumatic fever or heart murmur. The patient was in excellent health until 6 months ago when her symptoms developed; they have since become progressively worse. Physical examination reveals a well-developed, well-nourished, acyanotic woman who experiences mild respiratory distress at rest. The jugular pulse reveals large *a* waves. There is a prominent right ventricular heave. A palpable pulmonic closure is present and a grade III/VI systolic ejection murmur is heard at the left second intercostal space. A grade I/VI, blowing, holosystolic murmur is also noted at the lower left sternal border. The pulmonic closure is loud but splits normally with inspiration. The electrocardiogram reveals right ventricular hypertrophy. A chest x-ray shows dilation of the main pulmonary arteries with decreased vascularity in the outer one-third of the lung fields. The most likely diagnosis is which of the following?

(A) Atrial septal defect
(B) Ventricular septal defect
(C) Congenital pulmonic stenosis
(D) Tetralogy of Fallot
(E) Primary pulmonary hypertension

185. Cardiac auscultatory findings during normal pregnancy include all the following EXCEPT

(A) increase in intensity of the first heart sound
(B) persistent expiratory splitting of the second heart sound
(C) presence of a third heart sound
(D) presence of a fourth heart sound
(E) presence of a mammary souffle

186. In differentiating ventricular tachyarrhythmias from supraventricular tachyarrhythmias with aberrant ventricular conduction, findings that favor ventricular origin of the beats include all the following EXCEPT

(A) QRS duration exceeding 140 ms on scalar electrocardiogram
(B) fusion (Dressler) beats on rhythm strip
(C) AV dissociation on esophageal electrographic recording
(D) 2:1 AV block on cardiac monitor during carotid massage
(E) capture beats on cardiac rhythm strip

187. The rhythm strip displayed below reveals

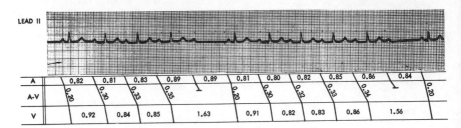

(A) atrial premature contractions
(B) junctional premature contractions
(C) AV dissociation
(D) type I second-degree AV block
(E) type II second-degree AV block

188. The electrocardiogram displayed below reveals which of the following patterns?

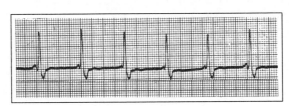

(A) Normal sinus rhythm
(B) Ventricular preexcitation
(C) Idioventricular rhythm
(D) Complete heart block
(E) Atrioventricular dissociation

189. A 43-year-old woman with a 1-year history of episodic leg edema and dyspnea is noted to have clubbing of the fingers. Her ECG is shown below. The correct diagnosis is

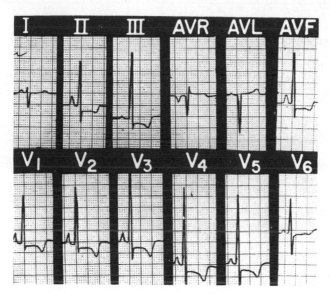

(A) inferior wall myocardial infarction
(B) right bundle branch block
(C) anterior wall myocardial infarction
(D) Wolff-Parkinson-White syndrome
(E) cor pulmonale

---

190. Which of the following statements correctly describes the most common primary cardiac tumor?

(A) The majority are located in the left ventricle
(B) It occurs more commonly in men than in women
(C) Clinical presentation usually mimics mitral valve disease
(D) It is histologically malignant
(E) Peak incidence occurs in the second decade of life

191. Warfarin (Coumadin) anticoagulation is used for a variety of cardiac conditions. Each of the following medications increases the anticoagulant effect of warfarin EXCEPT

(A) cimetidine
(B) rifampin
(C) quinidine
(D) α-methyldopa
(E) phenylbutazone

192. All the following statements concerning the rhythm strip displayed below are true EXCEPT

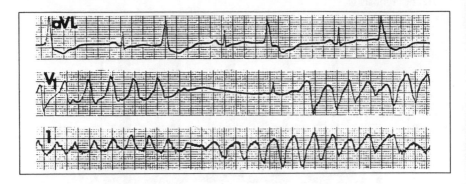

(A) it is usually initiated by a premature ventricular contraction in the presence of a long QT interval
(B) it most frequently results from drug administration
(C) once the arrhythmia is terminated by ventricular pacing, prophylaxis with quinidine is appropriate therapy
(D) it is associated with bradycardia, particularly when caused by AV block
(E) it may degenerate into ventricular fibrillation

---

193. The rhythm strip displayed below demonstrates

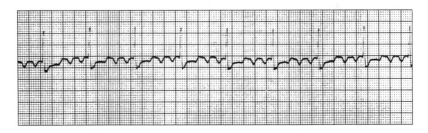

(A) normal sinus rhythm
(B) junctional rhythm
(C) atrial flutter with 4:1 atrioventricular block
(D) paroxysmal atrial tachycardia with 2:1 atrioventricular block
(E) complete heart block with 2:1 atrioventricular block

194. A 45-year-old white man is recovering from his first anterior myocardial infarction. As part of a program to control this patient's ischemic heart disease, his doctor discusses with the patient certain risk factors and how to avoid them. The physician would be justified in emphasizing all the following points EXCEPT that

(A) regular exercise can increase high-density lipoproteins, which are known to have a protective effect in ischemic heart disease

(B) scientific evidence conclusively demonstrates that stopping cigarette smoking decreases the risk of further complications of ischemic heart disease

(C) men with normal diastolic blood pressures (less than 83 mmHg) but elevated systolic blood pressures (greater than 158 mmHg) have in excess of a twofold increased risk of developing severe cardiovascular disease compared with persons with a normal systolic blood pressure

(D) the reduction to normal of diastolic blood pressures that lie between 95 and 105 mmHg has been clearly shown to reduce the risk of cardiovascular morbidity

(E) a family history of xanthomata is associated with an increased risk of ischemic heart disease

195. Mitral valve prolapse, the most common abnormality of human heart valves, is characterized by all the following statements EXCEPT

(A) migration of the systolic click and systolic murmur toward the first heart sound occurs during squatting

(B) echocardiography demonstrates systolic posterior motion of one or both mitral valve leaflets

(C) propranolol has been found to be helpful in those patients with palpitations and chest pain

(D) the syndrome appears to be inherited as an autosomal dominant condition with variable penetrance

(E) progression of the valvular defect to severe mitral regurgitation that necessitates surgical repair may occur

196. Digitalis glycosides are widely used in the treatment of heart failure and arrhythmias. Digoxin has a narrow toxic-therapeutic window, and in order to avoid digitalis intoxication, downward adjustment of digoxin dosage should be effected when it is given in conjunction with each of the following medications EXCEPT

(A) verapamil

(B) quinidine

(C) amiodarone

(D) erythromycin

(E) metoclopramide

197. The electrocardiogram displayed below is most compatible with which of the following diagnoses?

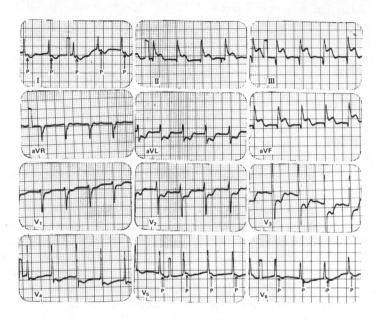

(A) Acute pericarditis with junctional tachycardia
(B) Acute anterior wall myocardial infarction with junctional tachycardia
(C) Acute inferior wall myocardial infarction with junctional tachycardia
(D) Acute inferior wall myocardial infarction with complete heart block
(E) Acute anterolateral myocardial infarction with junctional tachycardia

---

198. Each of the following cardiac conditions creates a relatively high risk of development of infective endocarditis EXCEPT

(A) coarctation of the aorta
(B) ventricular septal defect
(C) atrial septal defect
(D) prosthetic heart valve
(E) patent ductus arteriosus

199. All the following statements concerning the cardiac involvement in malignant carcinoid are true EXCEPT

(A) high cardiac output may occur
(B) a tendency toward pulmonic regurgitation is present
(C) the clinical syndrome is commonly that of tricuspid regurgitation
(D) serotonin antagonists do not affect progression of cardiac lesions
(E) valvular lesions occur only in the presence of hepatic metastases

200. A 54-year-old man is admitted to the coronary care unit for symptoms of retrosternal chest pressure, nausea, and intense diaphoresis. An electrocardiogram on admission is normal except for ST-segment elevation in leads V_1 to V_4. An electrocardiogram obtained the following day is shown below. Which of the following steps should next be taken in the management of this patient?

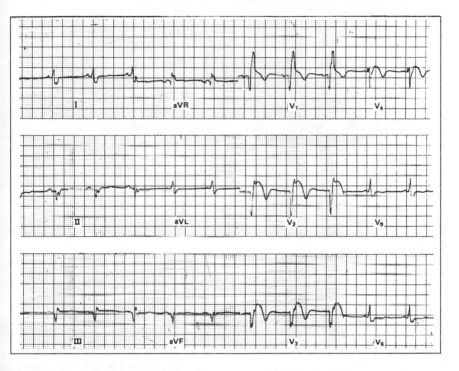

(A) Administration of heparin
(B) Administration of digitalis
(C) Administration of atropine
(D) Temporary transvenous pacing
(E) Observation alone

201. Each of the following statements pertaining to the coronary arterial circulation is correct EXCEPT

(A) the right coronary artery supplies the sinoatrial node in greater than 75 percent of patients
(B) the right coronary artery supplies the atrioventricular node in greater than 75 percent of patients
(C) the left circumflex coronary artery gives rise to obtuse marginal branches
(D) the left anterior descending artery gives rise to septal and diagonal branches
(E) the left anterior descending coronary artery arises from the left main coronary artery and courses along the anterior intraventricular groove

202. All the following statements regarding coarctation of the aorta are true EXCEPT that

(A) affected patients may complain of leg pain or fatigue
(B) it rarely produces symptoms of congestive heart failure in infancy
(C) it has a higher risk than normal of occurring in patients with Turner's syndrome
(D) it is commonly associated with aortic stenosis due to a bicuspid valve
(E) the lesion usually appears just distal to the left subclavian artery

203. Paradoxical splitting of the second heart sound may occur in association with each of the following cardiovascular disorders EXCEPT

(A) aortic stenosis
(B) right bundle branch block
(C) left bundle branch block
(D) left ventricular ischemia
(E) hypertension

204. A 50-year-old man with a long history of heavy cigarette smoking is admitted to a coronary care unit for an acute inferior wall myocardial infarction. Blood pressure on admission is 140/90 mmHg, pulse rate 80 beats per minute, and respiratory rate 16 breaths per minute. Examination reveals bibasilar rales and a loud S_4 gallop. The patient is given intravenous furosemide, 40 mg, and has a profound diuresis. Twelve hours later, his blood pressure is 80/60 mmHg and pulse rate 88 beats per minute, and he complains of retrosternal chest pain. A pulmonary artery catheter is inserted and the patient's pulmonary capillary wedge pressure is 4 mmHg. The most appropriate immediate therapy would be

(A) infusion of normal saline
(B) infusion of norepinephrine
(C) infusion of dopamine
(D) intravenous furosemide, 40 mg
(E) intravenous nitroglycerin

205. A syphilitic aneurysm of the aorta is most likely to occur at which of the following sites?

(A) Ascending aorta
(B) Aortic arch
(C) Descending thoracic aorta
(D) Abdominal aorta
(E) Bifurcation of the iliac arteries

206. A 45-year-old man is admitted to the hospital for an acute anterosep-tal myocardial infarction. Physical examination reveals a blood pressure of 150/100 mmHg and pulse of 100 beats per minute. The lung fields are clear and cardiac examination reveals only an S_4 gallop. Two days following admission, the patient develops severe shortness of breath. Blood pressure is 100/70 mmHg, pulse 120 beats per minute, and respiratory rate 32 breaths per minute. There are pulmonary rales bilaterally. A grade III/VI systolic murmur is heard at the lower left sternal border and both S_3 and S_4 gallops are present. The arterial P_{O_2} is 70 mmHg. The most likely diagnosis is

(A) pericardial effusion with tamponade
(B) papillary muscle dysfunction
(C) ruptured papillary muscle
(D) rupture of the interventricular septum
(E) acute pulmonary embolus

207. An 18-year-old man is involved in a street fight during which he sustains a severe knife wound to the chest. As a consequence of this injury, bleeding occurs into his pericardial cavity. He is placed on broad-spectrum antibiotic coverage that includes ampicillin and gentamicin. He makes a good recovery over the following month, but 3 months after the incident he suddenly becomes ill with a fever of 39.6°C (103.3°F). The symptoms and signs suggest pericarditis, pleuritis, and pneumonitis. In the 3 days that follow, the patient develops arthralgias, pericardial effusion, and leukocytosis. The most likely diagnosis is

(A) serum sickness induced by ampicillin
(B) rheumatoid arthritis
(C) Dressler's syndrome
(D) acute idiopathic pericarditis
(E) acute bacterial endocarditis

208. All the following statements regarding ventricular aneurysms are true EXCEPT

(A) they should be suspected in the presence of a persistent ST-segment elevation following a myocardial infarction
(B) they are more common with anterior than inferior wall myocardial infarctions
(C) risk of cardiac rupture is usually unrelated to reinfarction in the region
(D) recurrent arterial emboli may be the presenting sign
(E) the diagnosis may be suggested by the x-ray finding of calcium in the cardiac border

209. The rhythm strip displayed below reveals normal sinus rhythm with

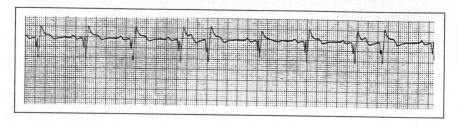

(A) periods of atrioventricular dissociation
(B) periods of Wenckebach atrioventricular block
(C) atrial premature contractions
(D) periods of complete heart block
(E) ventricular premature contractions

210. The rhythm strip (lead II) shown below was obtained from a patient who had severe obstructive lung disease. The strip most closely depicts which of the following arrhythmias?

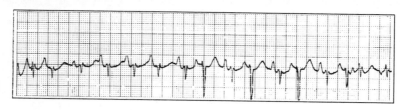

(A) Atrial flutter with varying atrioventricular block
(B) Atrial fibrillation
(C) Sinus tachycardia with premature ventricular contractions
(D) Atrioventricular dissociation
(E) Multifocal atrial tachycardia

211. A 75-year-old woman suffering from an acute anterior wall myocardial infarction is admitted to a coronary care unit. An ECG monitoring strip, obtained 6 h after admission, discloses the rhythm illustrated below. This rhythm probably represents

(A) rate-dependent left bundle branch block
(B) rate-dependent right bundle branch block
(C) complete heart block
(D) accelerated idioventricular rhythm
(E) junctional escape rhythm

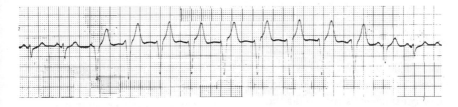

212. Hypertrophic cardiomyopathy is characterized by all the following statements EXCEPT that

(A) the carotid pulse of affected patients reveals a slow upstroke
(B) the associated murmur increases in the standing position
(C) a prominent fourth heart sound frequently occurs
(D) mitral regurgitation is present in 50 percent of affected patients
(E) beta blockers or calcium antagonists are useful for treating affected patients who have dyspnea or light-headedness

213. A 23-year-old woman with no previous history of cardiac disease develops symptoms and signs of acute bacterial endocarditis with mitral incompetence 1 week after an abortion. *Streptococcus faecalis* is grown in blood cultures. The most appropriate treatment for this patient would be

(A) mitral valve replacement followed by 6 weeks of antibiotic therapy
(B) parenteral administration of ampicillin, 12 g daily for 4 weeks
(C) parenteral administration of penicillin G, 24 million units per day for 6 weeks
(D) parenteral administration of ampicillin, 12 g daily, and gentamicin, 3 mg/kg daily, for 4 weeks
(E) parenteral administration of vancomycin, 1 g daily for 4 weeks, with streptomycin, 1 g daily added to the protocol for the first 2 weeks

DIRECTIONS: Each question below contains four suggested responses of which **one or more** is correct. Select

A	if	**1, 2, and 3**	are correct
B	if	**1 and 3**	are correct
C	if	**2 and 4**	are correct
D	if	**4**	is correct
E	if	**1, 2, 3, and 4**	are correct

214. A 54-year-old man with a history of viral pericarditis is found on physical examination to have hepatomegaly and distended neck veins; chest x-rays reveal calcification of the pericardium. Correct statements concerning this patient's condition include which of the following?

(1) Episodes of acute pulmonary edema punctuate the clinical course

(2) It may be complicated by a protein-losing gastroenteropathy

(3) A paradoxical pulse is an uncommon finding

(4) Echocardiography demonstrates paradoxical septal motion

215. A patient with a congenital bicuspid valve develops auscultatory evidence of aortic regurgitation. True statements regarding this condition include which of the following?

(1) Chronic aortic regurgitation of mild to moderate severity is characterized by a long asymptomatic phase

(2) Development of symptoms of congestive heart failure in aortic regurgitation heralds rapid clinical deterioration

(3) Symptomatic patients with evidence of left ventricular dysfunction at rest should be advised to have valve surgery

(4) Asymptomatic patients with evidence of left ventricular dysfunction at rest should be advised to have surgery

216. Fluid in the pericardial space exceeding the 20 mL of volume normally present may result in cardiac tamponade. Characteristic findings associated with this clinical entity include which of the following?

(1) Loss of the y descent and accentuation of the x descent on the right atrial pressure waveform

(2) Inspiratory rise in arterial systolic pressure

(3) Tachycardia and narrow pulse pressure

(4) Inspiratory increase in jugular venous pressure (Kussmaul's sign)

DIRECTIONS: Each group of questions below consists of lettered headings followed by a set of numbered items. For each numbered item select the **one** lettered heading with which it is **most** closely associated. Each lettered heading may be used **once, more than once, or not at all.**

Questions 217–219

For each cardiac disorder below, select the clinical finding with which it is most closely associated.

(A) Sharp y descent in jugular pulse tracing
(B) Middiastolic rumble at apex
(C) Large v waves in jugular pulse tracing
(D) Slow y descent in jugular pulse tracing
(E) Prominent c waves in jugular pulse tracing

217. Tricuspid stenosis

218. Aortic regurgitation

219. Constrictive pericarditis

Questions 220-223

Match the agents below with associated side effects.

(A) Increased triglyceride levels
(B) Volume retention
(C) Lupus-like syndrome
(D) Nephrotic syndrome
(E) Gynecomastia

220. Captopril

221. Hydralazine

222. Propranolol

223. Minoxidil

Questions 224–227

For each electrolyte abnormality below, select the electrocardiographic picture with which it is most commonly associated.

(A) No known electrocardiographic abnormalities
(B) Prolonged QT interval
(C) Short QT interval
(D) Widened QRS complex
(E) Prominent U waves

224. Hypokalemia

225. Hyperkalemia

226. Hypocalcemia

227. Hyponatremia

Questions 228-230

Match the following.

(A) Bronchiectasis
(B) Coarctation of the aorta
(C) Ventricular septal defect
(D) Homocystinuria
(E) None of the above

228. Dextrocardia

229. Dilatation of aortic and pulmonary arteries

230. Hyperextensible joints

Questions 231–235

A normal jugular venous pulse wave in relation to first and second heart sounds is displayed below. For each cardiac phenomenon described, select the segment of the venous pulse wave with which it is most likely to be associated.

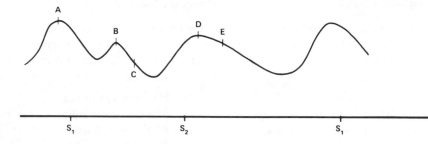

231. Atrial contraction

232. Filling of right atrium while tricuspid valve is closed

233. Opening of tricuspid valve

234. Bulging of tricuspid valve into right atrium

235. S_4 gallop

Questions 236–239

Match the definitions below with the appropriate terms related to probability analysis.

(A) Sensitivity
(B) Specificity
(C) Positive predictive value
(D) Negative predictive value
(E) None of the above

236. True positives divided by true positives plus false positives

237. True positives divided by true positives plus false negatives

238. True negatives divided by true negatives plus false negatives

239. True negatives divided by true negatives plus false positives

Questions 240–243

Match each pulse pattern with the correct disorder.

(A) Hypertrophic obstructive cardiomyopathy
(B) Dilated cardiomyopathy
(C) Cardiac tamponade
(D) Aortic stenosis
(E) None of the above

240. Pulsus parvus et tardus

241. Pulsus alternans

242. Pulsus paradoxus

243. Pulsus bisferiens

Cardiology

Answers

182. The answer is E. *(Houston, Am Heart J 117:911, 1989.)* There has been a decline in age-adjusted death rates from cerebrovascular accident, coronary heart disease (CHD), and all cardiovascular diseases since 1968 in the United States. It is believed that the reduction in CHD mortality is mainly due to reduction in the risk factors of CHD and out-of-hospital as well as in-hospital survival of patients with acute myocardial infarction. Antihypertensive drug therapy of patients with diastolic pressures equal to or greater than 110 mmHg has been shown to reduce the incidence of CHD. However, pharmacotherapeutic treatment of mild hypertension (diastolic blood pressure 90 to 105 mmHg) has not demonstrated favorable effects on the morbidity and mortality of CHD, possibly as a result of unfavorable effects of antihypertensive medications on other CHD risk factors, such as lipids and glucose.

183. The answer is C. *(Braunwald, ed 3. pp 666–667, 888–889. Hurst, ed 7. pp 588–589.)* Hypersensitive carotid sinus syndrome is a condition in which stimulation of the carotid sinus results in ventricular asystole caused by sinus arrest or sinoatrial block, or hypotension caused by vasodilatation, or both. The absence of atrial activity probably masks transient coexistent atrioventricular (AV) block. The absence of junctional or ventricular escape rhythms in some patients suggests the influence of enhanced vagal tone on these subsidiary pacemakers as well. The postulated mechanism for the carotid sinus reflex involves pressure-sensitive receptors in the adventitia of the carotid artery, afferent neural traffic via the glossopharyngeal nerve or other routes through cervical sympathetics through the twelfth cranial nerve, and efferent innervation via the vagus nerve and sympathetics. It is believed that the vagus nerve is responsible for the cardioinhibitory component, while sympathetic fibers mediate inhibition of arterial vasoconstriction and possible cholinergic vasodilator activity. Although atropine transiently blocks cardioinhibitory carotid sinus hypersensitivity, permanent pacemaker implantation is often necessary for recurrent episodes. Because of the likelihood of coexistent AV block during episodes, a ventricular or AV sequential pacemaker should be used. The vasodepressor form, as well as the mixed vasodepressor and cardioinhibitory form of this syndrome, is especially difficult to treat. Patients should be instructed to avoid any activities that may exert pressure on the carotid sinus. Medications that may accentuate carotid sinus hypersensitivity (including beta-adrenergic blocking agents, digitalis glycosides, α-methyldopa, and clonidine) should be withdrawn. Pharmacotherapy with anticholinergic and sympathomimetic agents may be effective in controlling symptoms when avoidance of carotid sinus stimulation and administration of medications is unsuccessful in preventing episodes of syncope. Additional measures, including surgical denervation or radiotherapy ablation of the carotid sinus nerve, may be undertaken. Since mixed cardioinhibitory and vasodepressor carotid sinus hypersensitivity will often coexist, a pronounced vasodepressor component with recurrent syncope may manifest itself despite permanent pacemaker implantation.

184. The answer is E. *(Braunwald, ed 3. pp 805–813. Hurst, ed 7. pp 1198–1202.)* In the patient presented in the question, the absence of a history of heart murmur makes congenital heart disease an unlikely diagnosis. The rapid onset of the symptoms described makes primary pulmonary hypertension the most likely cause. While its cause is unknown, the basic pathology of this disease involves thickening of the walls of the pulmonary arterioles resulting in progressive resistance to blood flow through the lungs. As the disease progresses, pulmonary blood flow and cardiac output are reduced and show little increase during exertion. Primary pulmonary hypertension tends to have a peak incidence in young women. Death usually occurs within 4 to 5 years after onset of symptoms. Affected patients characteristically have the symptom complex and physical findings described in the question. Systolic ejection murmurs in the pulmonic area result from ejection of blood into a proximally dilated pulmonary artery. Holosystolic murmurs at the lower left sternal border probably represent tricuspid insufficiency from right ventricular enlargement. Dilatation of the proximal portion of the pulmonary arteries, with decreased blood flow to the outer third of the lung fields, is a further indication of pulmonary hypertension.

185. The answer is D. *(Braunwald, ed 3. p 1852.)* Cardiac auscultatory findings of pregnancy begin in the first trimester and generally disappear within the first few days after parturition. Increase in heart rate and ventricular contractility result in increased amplitude of the first heart sound. The second heart sound demonstrates persistent expiratory splitting, especially during the third trimester. Third heart sounds, which are common in the young, increase in intensity during pregnancy as a result of increased rate and flow. Healthy young women do not have fourth heart sounds during normal pregnancy. Innocent midsystolic murmurs, which originate from flow in pulmonary and brachiocephalic arteries, increase in intensity owing to increased cardiac output and stroke volume during gestation. The mammary souffle is a systolic or continuous murmur heard over the breasts in late pregnancy and in the postpartum lactating woman. The murmurs of mitral, aortic, or pulmonic stenosis increase in intensity because of increased blood flow and shortening of diastolic filling time. Murmurs of mitral and aortic regurgitation may decrease in intensity as the systemic vascular resistance falls during pregnancy. The systolic murmurs of mitral valve prolapse and hypertrophic cardiomyopathy may decrease in amplitude because of increasing left ventricular volume during pregnancy.

186.   The answer is D. *(Braunwald, ed 3. p 702. Hurst, ed 7. pp 517–519. Wellens, Am J Med 64:27, 1978.)* While QRS duration less than 120 ms strongly favors supraventricular origin of cardiac rhythm, no similar feature as accurately predicts ventricular origin. While QRS duration of greater than 140 ms strongly supports the diagnosis of ventricular origin, aberrant conduction of supraventricular beats may exceed this duration as well. AV dissociation similarly favors ventricular origin; however, AV junctional tachycardias without retrograde conduction (allowing independent atrial activity) may occur. Fusion and capture beats strongly favor ventricular origin, although varying degrees of fusion of two supraventricular impulses may also occur. AV block induced by carotid massage suggests that ventricular activation is dependent on atrial discharge and supports supraventricular origin of the rhythm.

187.   The answer is D. *(Hurst, ed 7. pp 523–525.)* Type I second-degree AV block, the more common of the two forms of second-degree AV block, is characterized by the following: (1) after progressive lengthening of the PR interval, the final P wave is not followed by a QRS complex, (2) the increment by which the PR interval increases progressively decreases, and (3) the RR interval containing the dropped beat is less than two times the shortest preceding RR interval. Type I second-degree AV block is usually due to a conduction delay within the AV node.

188.   The answer is E. *(Braunwald, ed 3. pp 707–708. Mandel, ed 2. pp 241–253.)* The rhythm strip exhibited both in the question and below reveals a P wave before the first QRS complex, with a short PR interval. The P waves then move into the QRS complexes until the end of the strip, where a P wave is again seen preceding a QRS complex. This strip reveals atrioventricular (AV) dissociation in which the atria are being depolarized by the sinus node and the ventricles are being depolarized by a junctional or AV nodal focus. This particular example of AV dissociation is termed *isorhythmic dissociation* since the rates of atria and ventricles are almost equal. The preferred meaning of AV dissociation implies two separate pacemakers, with the lower focus faster in rate than the higher focus. This situation differs from complete heart block, in which the rate of the lower focus (an escape rhythm) is slower than the higher. In AV dissociation, the lower focus is firing faster than the higher because of increased automaticity and thus controls the ventricles. AV dissociation is commonly associated with digitalis toxicity and inferior wall myocardial infarction.

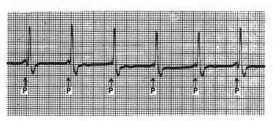

189.   The answer is E. *(Hurst, ed 7. pp 1220–1226.)* Cor pulmonale is characterized by the presence of pulmonary hypertension and consequent right ventricular
dysfunction. Its causes include diseases leading to hypoxic vasoconstriction, as in
cystic fibrosis; occlusion of the pulmonary vasculature, as in pulmonary thrombo-
embolism; and parenchymal destruction, as in sarcoidosis. The right ventricle, in the
presence of a chronic increase in afterload, becomes hypertrophic, dilates, and fails.
The electrocardiographic findings, as illustrated in the question, include tall, peaked
P waves in leads II, III, and aVF, which indicate right atrial enlargement; tall R
waves in leads V_1 to V_3 and a deep S wave in V_6 with associated ST-T wave
changes, which indicate right ventricular hypertrophy; and right axis deviation.
Right bundle branch block occurs in 15 percent of patients.

190.   The answer is C. *(Braunwald, ed 3. pp 1470–1475.)* Myxomas are histologically benign and account for up to one-half of all cases of primary cardiac
tumors. Because they are most commonly located in the left atrium and are peduncu-
lated, they are particularly prone to mimicking mitral stenosis as a result of a
ball-valve effect and causing mitral regurgitation due to trauma to the mitral
leaflets. Noncardiac manifestations of myxomas include fever, weight loss, arthralgia, and anemia. Surgical excision is curative. Cardiac sarcomas are the most
common malignant primary cardiac tumor and are uniformly rapidly fatal.

191.   The answer is B. *(Braunwald, ed 3. p 1774.)* A variety of pharmacotherapeutic agents affect the anticoagulant effect of warfarin. Some compete for
albumin binding, which displaces warfarin from the blood and increases its delivery
to the liver for excretion. Other drugs increase microsomal enzyme activity, thereby
enhancing drug metabolism. Finally, others impair intestinal absorption of the drug.
Drugs that increase the anticoagulant effect of warfarin include certain antibiotics,
α-methyldopa, cimetidine, quinidine, anabolic steroids, phenylbutazone, D-
thyroxine, sulfinpyrazone, and clofibrate. Drugs that decrease the anticoagulant
effect of warfarin include vitamin K, antihistamines, certain antacids, rifampin,
cholestyramine, barbiturates, and griseofulvin. In addition, metabolic and dietary
influences that change the disposition of albumin and vitamin K alter the anticoagulant effect of warfarin as well.

192.   The answer is C. *(Braunwald, ed 3. pp 698–700. Somberg, Am Heart J
111:1162–1176, 1986.)* Torsades de pointes is a rapid ventricular tachycardia
characterized by unusual QRS complexes whose axes shift back and forth around
the baseline. It occurs most commonly in patients who have prolonged QT intervals.
Indeed, any influence that prolongs the QT interval—such as quinidine, procain-
amide, tricyclic antidepressants, phenothiazines, hypokalemia, or hypocalcemia—or
congenital QT prolongation may cause torsades. This rhythm is clinically important
because it may degenerate to ventricular fibrillation, and it should not be treated
with QT-lengthening antiarrhythmics. Emergent therapy may include either

ventricular pacing or isoproterenol infusion along with correction of the underlying abnormality in the acquired forms or with the addition of drugs that shorten the QT interval (such as phenytoin and beta blockers) in the congenital varieties. For patients with recurrent symptomatic torsades despite maximal medical therapy, left-sided cervicothoracic sympathetic ganglionectomy may be effective. If this surgery is also ineffective in preventing symptomatic arrhythmias, implantation of an automatic cardioverter-defibrillator should be considered.

193. The answer is C. *(Braunwald, ed 3. pp 671–672. Mandel, ed 2. pp 228–230.)* The rhythm strip exhibited in the question reveals atrial flutter with 4:1 atrioventricular (AV) block. Atrial flutter is characterized by an atrial rate of 280 to 320 per minute; the electrocardiogram typically reveals a sawtooth baseline configuration due to the flutter waves. In the strip presented, every fourth atrial depolarization is conducted through the AV node, resulting in a ventricular rate of 75 per minute.

194. The answer is D. *(Braunwald, ed 3. pp 862–865, 1173–1174.)* To date, reduction of excessive cardiovascular morbidity has been demonstrated clearly only in patients whose diastolic pressures had exceeded 105 mmHg. There is a growing consensus among cardiologists, however, that the diastolic pressure should be kept at, or below, 90 mmHg. Excellent evidence now suggests that high-density lipoproteins protect against the development of atherosclerosis. A decrease in cigarette smoking and the undertaking of regular exercise both raise the circulating level of high-density lipoproteins. Epidemiologic studies have conclusively demonstrated the benefit of stopping cigarette smoking, as well as the dangers of smoking. Elevations in systolic blood pressure, diastolic blood pressure, or both are clearly associated with an increased risk of cardiovascular disease.

195. The answer is A. *(Braunwald, ed 3. pp 1045–1051.)* The fundamental defect in mitral valve prolapse is an abnormality of the valve's connective tissue with secondary proliferation of myxomatous tissue. The redundant leaflet or leaflets prolapse toward the left atrium in systole, which results in the auscultated click and murmur and characteristic echocardiographic findings. Any maneuver that reduces left ventricular size, such as standing or Valsalva, allows the click and murmur to occur earlier in systole; conversely, those maneuvers that increase left ventricular size, such as squatting and propranolol administration, delay the onset of the click and murmur. While most patients with mitral valve prolapse have a benign prognosis, a small percentage die suddenly. Antibiotic prophylaxis to prevent endocarditis is recommended for those with typical auscultatory findings, including a systolic murmur.

196. The answer is E. *(Braunwald, ed 3. pp 500–501. Hurst, ed 7. pp 1755–1758.)* Drugs interact with digoxin by a variety of mechanisms. Verapamil decreases renal and total body clearance of digoxin and results in approximately a 70 to 100 percent increase in steady-state serum digoxin levels; verapamil thus requires a decrease in digoxin dose by approximately one-half. Quinidine increases absorption, decreases volume of distribution, and decreases renal and total body clearance of digoxin. The result is approximately a 100 percent increase in steady-state serum digoxin level, which requires a decrease in digoxin dosage by approximately one-half. Amiodarone decreases renal and total body clearance of digoxin and increases steady-state serum digoxin levels by 70 to 100 percent; it likewise requires a decrease in digoxine dosage by one-half. Erythromycin increases the bioavailability of digoxin by decreasing intestinal metabolism of digoxin by certain gut flora; the result is a 43 to 150 percent increase in steady-state digoxin levels. Metoclopramide decreased bioavailability of digoxin by increasing intestinal motility, which results in a 25 to 36 percent drop in steady-state digitalis levels. Other medications that decrease serum digoxin levels include cholestyramine, certain antacids, neomycin, and sulfasalazine.

197. The answer is C. *(Braunwald, ed 3. pp 203–214, 1262–1272, 1286–1287. Mandel, ed 2. pp 261–263.)* The electrocardiogram presented in the question demonstrates an acute inferior wall myocardial infarction with ST-segment elevation in leads II, III, and a VF. The ST-segment depressions seen in the majority of the other leads are probably reciprocal changes to the ST-segment elevations mentioned. The ST-segment elevation of acute pericarditis, however, is not accompanied by reciprocal changes. Close examination of the tracing reveals P waves following each QRS complex. Whether the P wave precedes, is buried within, or follows the QRS complex in a junctional rhythm depends upon the location of the ectopic focus in the atrioventricular (AV) node and the rates of antegrade and retrograde conduction. In this example, the ectopic focus in the AV node reaches the ventricle just before it reaches the atrium, resulting in the P wave following the QRS complex. Junctional tachycardia is diagnosed when the rate of the pacemaker in the AV node exceeds 60 per minute. Common causes of this arrhythmia are inferior wall myocardial infarction, digitalis intoxication, and myocarditis.

198. The answer is C. *(Hurst, ed 7. p 732.)* The list of conditions at relatively high risk of development of infective endocarditis includes Marfan's syndrome, prosthetic heart valves, coarctation of the aorta, aortic valve disease, ventricular septal defect, mitral insufficiency, and patent ductus arteriosus. Mitral valve prolapse, pure mitral stenosis, and tricuspid and pulmonary valve disease are among the conditions at intermediate risk. Among the conditions considered to be at very low risk are atrial septal defect, syphilitic aortitis, and cardiac pacemakers.

199. The answer is B. *(Braunwald, ed 3. pp 1439–1440.)* Tumors producing the carcinoid syndrome are slowly growing neoplasms arising from the gastrointestinal tract or derivatives of the embryonic foregut, testes, and ovaries. Their clinical features include cutaneous flushing, telangiectasis, intestinal hypermotility, bronchospasm, and evidence of valvular heart disease. The right side of the heart is more commonly involved than the left and there is a tendency of developing tricuspid regurgitation and pulmonic stenosis with consequent right-sided heart failure. The morbidity from these tumors results largely from their variable expression of serotonin, histamine, substance P, and bradykinin. While no effective antitumor regimen exists, therapy of heart failure (using digitalis and diuretics), vasomotor symptoms (using histamine and serotonin antagonists), and serious valvular dysfunction (by valvulotomy or replacement) may be employed.

200. The answer is D. *(Braunwald, ed 3. pp 1266-1267. Mandel, ed 2. pp 102-105.)* The electrocardiogram shown in the question reveals an evolving anteroseptal myocardial infarction. There is ST-segment elevation in leads V_1 to V_3. Right bundle branch block (RBBB) is present with QRS duration of 0.12 s wide and terminal S waves in leads I, aVL, and V_6. The classic rSR′ of RBBB is not seen since the initial R wave in V_1 has been replaced with a Q wave as a result of the anterior infarction. The electrocardiogram also reveals marked left axis deviation consistent with a left anterior hemiblock. Since both the right bundle and the anterior division of the left bundle are damaged as a result of the infarction, conduction to the ventricles is dependent solely on the posterior division of the left bundle. In the presence of an acute anteroseptal myocardial infarction, with new bifasicular block, temporary transvenous pacing is indicated as a prophylactic measure in case complete heart block develops.

201. The answer is A. *(Braunwald, ed 3. pp 272-275.)* The right coronary artery supplies the sinoatrial node in approximately 50 to 60 percent of cases and the atrioventricular node in approximately 77 to 90 percent of cases. The left anterior descending coronary artery arises from the left main coronary artery and courses along the anterior interventricular sulcus toward the cardiac apex. Along its course it gives rise to septal branches, which perfuse the interventricular septum, and diagonal branches, which perfuse the anterolateral aspect of the heart. The left circumflex coronary artery arises from the left main coronary artery and courses along the left atrioventricular sulcus; it gives rise to obtuse marginal branches, which perfuse the lateral aspect of the left ventricle. The right coronary artery arises from the right aortic sinus and courses along the right atrioventricular sulcus; it gives rise to acute marginal branches and posterior left ventricular branches. The dominant coronary artery (the right coronary artery in 77 to 90 percent of cases and the left circumflex in the remainder) supplies the diaphragmatic portion of the left ventricle and the inferior portion of the interventricular septum.

202. The answer is B. *(Braunwald, ed 3. pp 994-997.)* Coarctation of the aorta is a congenital abnormality characterized by a region of narrowed aorta; 95 percent of these lesions occur just distal to the left subclavian artery. Because of decreased blood flow to the lower extremities, affected patients may complain of leg fatigue or pain on exertion. A congenital bicuspid aortic valve occurs concomitantly with coarctation in approximately 50 percent of such people. Symptoms of congestive heart failure are common in infants who have coarctation and usually appear in the first months of life. Patients afflicted with Turner's syndrome have a high incidence of aortic coarctation.

203. The answer is B. *(Hurst, ed 7. pp 193–194.)* Normally, the second heart sound (S_2) is composed of aortic closure followed by pulmonic closure. Because inspiration increases blood return to the right side of the heart, pulmonic closure is delayed, which results in normal splitting of S_2 during inspiration. Paradoxical splitting of S_2, however, refers to a splitting of S_2 that is narrowed instead of widened with inspiration consequent to a delayed aortic closure. Paradoxical splitting can result from any electrical or mechanical event that delays left ventricular systole. Thus, aortic stenosis and hypertension, which increase resistance to systolic ejection of blood, delay closure of the aortic valve. Acute ischemia from angina or acute myocardial infarction also can delay ejection of blood from the left ventricle. The most common cause of paradoxical splitting—left bundle branch block—delays electrical activation of the left ventricle. Right bundle branch block results in a wide splitting of S_2 that widens further during inspiration.

204. The answer is A. *(Braunwald, ed 3. pp 1273–1275. Forrester, N Engl J Med 295:1356–1360, 1976.)* The pulmonary artery catheter provides an accurate bedside means of determining left ventricular filling pressures. The catheter is passed through a vein to the heart where it is placed in a pulmonary artery. When the balloon at the tip is inflated, the catheter records pulmonary capillary wedge pressure, which is equivalent to left atrial pressure and, in the absence of mitral stenosis, to left ventricular diastolic pressure. The level of pulmonary capillary wedge pressure correlates with left ventricular volume. Normal pulmonary capillary pressure is 5 to 12 mmHg. Levels above 18 to 20 mmHg are associated with signs of congestive heart failure. On admission to the hospital, the patient had bibasilar rales, which may have represented pulmonary disease, since an S_3 gallop, which would have suggested congestive failure, was not heard. His postdiuresis pulmonary capillary pressure of 4 mmHg is low and suggests hypovolemia. Appropriate therapy for this patient would be to administer intravenous saline to bring his pulmonary capillary pressures up to at least 12 mmHg.

205. The answer is A. *(Braunwald, ed 3. pp 1566–1568.)* Aneurysms of the aorta from syphilis occur most commonly in the ascending aorta and least commonly in the descending thoracic or abdominal aorta. Calcification in the wall of the ascending aorta is frequently present. Aneurysm formation occurs 15 to 30 years following infection with syphilis. Aortic valvular insufficiency is the most common complication of syphilitic aortitis. In addition, the coronary ostia may be involved, resulting in angina or myocardial infarction.

206. The answer is D. *(Braunwald, ed 3. pp 1283-1284. Hurst, ed 7. pp 1070-1071, 2221-2222.)* The most likely diagnoses in any patient suffering acute myocardial infarction who develops a new murmur and severe congestive failure are ventricular septal defect (VSD) and papillary muscle dysfunction (PMD). The murmur of acquired VSD following infarction tends to be maximal at the lower sternal border and may be associated with a thrill. Mitral regurgitation due to PMD is usually maximal at the apex. However, it is sometimes very difficult to determine by examination alone exactly which defect is present. Doppler echocardiography and right-heart catheterization are useful procedures to differentiate VSD from PMD. Rupture of a papillary muscle is a catastrophic event associated with shock and intractable pulmonary edema. The hypoxemia exhibited by the patient presented in the question, while suggestive of pulmonary embolism, is compatible with severe congestive failure alone.

207. The answer is C. *(Braunwald, ed 3. pp 1287, 1521-1523.)* Dressler's syndrome may develop following the escape of blood into the pericardial cavity from a variety of causes (e.g., cardiac surgery, myocardial infarction, trauma to the heart from a nonpenetrating blow to the chest, perforation of the heart by a pacemaker catheter). The syndrome usually occurs 2 to 4 weeks following the cardiac injury but quite frequently appears after a lapse of months, even years. Relapses are very common. Symptoms of Dressler's syndrome include fever, pleuritis, pericarditis, pneumonitis, arthritis, and leukocytosis. The syndrome, which is thought to be a result of immunologic sensitization to cardiac antigens presented to lymphocytes at the time of the injury, correlates with the presence of antimyocardial antibodies; the clinical picture associated with the syndrome resembles that seen with both viral and idiopathic pericarditis. In the patient presented, the history of a knife wound helps make these entities less likely as diagnostic possibilities. In mild cases, no treatment other than analgesics is needed. Dressler's syndrome can be very serious and even fatal. Severe cases usually respond to corticosteroids. The age and sex of this particular patient make a diagnosis of rheumatoid arthritis unlikely. While pleural effusions are relatively common in rheumatoid arthritis, pericardial effusions are rare. Bacterial endocarditis could be associated with all the patient's symptoms, but clear evidence of endocardial disease would be required to support such a diagnosis.

208. The answer is C. *(Hurst, ed 7. pp 932-934, 1073.)* The formation of a ventricular aneurysm is a late complication of myocardial infarction and the diagnosis is suggested by the presence of persistent ST-segment elevation several months after the infarction. Patients who have an aneurysm may present with arterial emboli, recurrent ventricular arrhythmias, or intractable congestive heart failure. Rupture is extremely unlikely unless there is a reinfarction over the same involved area of the ventricle. The chest x-ray occasionally reveals calcium in the wall of the aneurysm or in a mural thrombus within the aneurysm.

209.   The answer is C. *(Braunwald, ed 3. pp 669–671. Mandel, ed 2. pp 187, 199.)* The rhythm strip shown below, and in the question, demonstrates normal sinus rhythm with two atrial premature contractions (beats numbered 5 and 9). P waves of atrial premature contractions appear earlier than expected and differ in morphology from the P waves of the sinus beats. They may be conducted to the ventricles resulting in relatively normal-appearing QRS complexes or, if they occur during the refractory period of the atrioventricular node or the ventricles, they may be blocked. In that situation, premature P waves would differ in morphology from the P waves of the sinus beats and no QRS complex would follow the premature P wave.

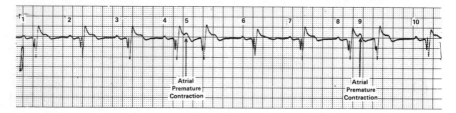

210.   The answer is E. *(Braunwald, ed 3. pp 496–497, 541. Mandel, ed 2. pp 224, 226, 228.)* Multifocal atrial tachycardia tends to occur in patients who have severe lung disease. It is characterized by varying P-wave morphology and PR intervals. The rhythm strip shown below exhibits at least three different P-wave shapes. The beats numbered 8, 10, and 12 are probably aberrantly conducted, resulting in their more bizarre appearance. The presence of severe pulmonary disease in the patient from whom the strip was obtained is suggested by the tall, peaked P waves (P pulmonale).

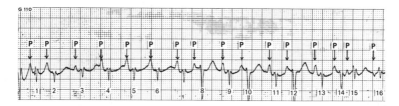

211.   The answer is D. *(Braunwald, ed 3. pp 194–202, 698. Hurst, ed 7. pp 512–515.)* The ECG strip presented in the question demonstrates normal sinus rhythm with a period of accelerated idioventricular rhythm (AIVR). AIVR is due to increased automaticity and usually is associated with acute myocardial infarction or digitalis intoxication. On the ECG, the rate of the AIVR is slightly faster than that of the first two sinus beats. Beats numbered 3 and 12 represent fusion beats since the

QRS configuration is intermediate between that of the sinus beats and those of AIVR. Characteristics of this arrhythmia are the wide, bizarre complexes suggesting ventricular origin, the presence of fusion beats, and rates up to 120 beats per minute. Rate-dependent left or right bundle branch block is characterized by widening of the QRS complex, but each complex is preceded by a P wave with a constant PR interval. In complete heart block, P waves are independent of and occur at a rate faster than the QRS complexes. Junctional escape rhythms most commonly occur at rates of 30 to 60 beats per minute and the QRS complexes are usually normal in configuration.

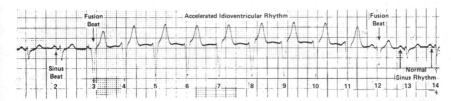

212. The answer is A. *(Braunwald, ed 3. pp 1418–1430.)* Hypertrophic cardiomyopathy is characterized by thickening of the muscular interventricular septum resulting in obstruction to left ventricular ejection of blood during ventricular systole and impairment of left ventricular filling during diastole. The typical murmur is a systolic ejection murmur along the left sternal border. Any maneuver that increases left ventricular volume will decrease the obstruction and murmur. Conversely, standing, which causes venous pooling in the lower extremities, will decrease ventricular volume and thus cause the obstruction and murmur to increase. The arterial pulse has a typical brisk upstroke and may display two palpable peaks in the pulse wave. A loud fourth heart sound is common and results from the blood from atrial systole encountering a thick, noncompliant ventricle. Associated systolic anterior motion of the anterior leaflet of the mitral valve causes mitral regurgitation in 50 percent of patients. Beta blockers or calcium antagonists, by affecting hypercontractile systolic function and abnormal diastolic filling, may relieve symptoms like dyspnea on exertion, chest pain, or light-headedness.

213. The answer is D. *(Braunwald, ed 3. pp 1102–1103. Hurst, ed 7. pp 1248–1251.)* In contrast to subacute bacterial endocarditis, acute bacterial endocarditis frequently develops on normal heart valves. Although endocardial destruction at times may be so severe and so rapid that emergency surgery is necessary, often positive blood cultures will allow antibiotic therapy to be successfully introduced and surgery avoided. In genitourinary infections, the invading organisms often are enterococci (*Streptococcus faecalis, S. faecium*). Because these microorganisms are relatively resistant to penicillin, a combination of ampicillin and gentamicin, acting synergistically against enterococci, is recommended. A daily regimen of 12 g of ampicillin and 3 mg/kg of gentamicin for 4 weeks will usually suffice.

When acute bacterial endocarditis is caused by group D nonenterococcal organisms such as *S. bovis*, penicillin alone is quite satisfactory. An additional advantage of penicillin is the avoidance of the potential toxic effects of gentamicin. In either situation, parenteral treatment must continue for a minimum of 4 weeks. In patients who are allergic to penicillin, vancomycin and streptomycin are recommended.

214. The answer is C (2, 4). *(Braunwald, ed 3. pp 501–508.)* Constrictive pericarditis may follow almost any insult to the pericardium and is characterized by an obliteration of the pericardial cavity with consequent constriction of the heart and restriction of ventricular filling. Causes include trauma, infection, neoplasia, radiation, uremia, and connective tissue diseases; in many cases, no inciting event can be determined. The basic defect in this condition is an impairment of diastolic filling and a decrease in stroke volume; cardiac systolic function may be normal. Patients typically present with fatigue and dyspnea on exertion; acute pulmonary edema is uncommon. Symptoms and signs of right-sided heart failure are present and include hepatomegaly, ascites, impaired lymphatic drainage from the small intestine leading to a protein-losing state, and dependent edema. A paradoxical pulse is found in one-third of patients and may be associated with Kussmaul's sign. Echocardiography demonstrates pericardial thickening and paradoxical septal motion in patients with constrictive pericarditis. Treatment involves surgical resection of the pericardium.

215. The answer is E (all). *(Hoshino, Arch Intern Med 146:349–352, 1986. Hurst, ed 7. pp 805–816.)* Chronic aortic regurgitation generally progresses slowly with very low mortality during a long asymptomatic phase. Indeed, approximately 90 percent of patients with mild-to-moderate aortic insufficiency will survive for a decade. Once symptoms develop, however, there is rapid clinical deterioration associated with gross left ventricular enlargement and depressed myocardial contractility. Average survival of patients is 5 years after onset of angina and 2 years after onset of congestive heart failure. Furthermore, preoperative ventricular function is a strong predictor of survival (ejection fraction ≥ 45 percent and a cardiac index > 2.5 L/min/m^2 are associated with a higher postoperative survival). Because prognosis is related to ventricular function, symptomatic patients and asymptomatic patients with evidence of left ventricular dysfunction at rest as measured by radionuclide studies or echocardiography should have surgery. Asymptomatic patients with normal left ventricular function at rest and documented left ventricular dysfunction on exertion should be advised to have surgery as well.

216. The answer is B (1, 3). *(Hurst, ed 7. pp 1354–1362. Rackley, pp 181–191.)* Cardiac tamponade is characterized by a rise in intrapericardial pressure sufficient to cause a decrease in cardiac filling, a reduction in cardiac output, and peripheral hypoperfusion. Causes include trauma, malignancy (most commonly lung and breast cancers), infection, uremia, connective tissue diseases, and radiation therapy. Patients present with symptoms of visceral and hepatic congestion, dyspnea, and chest discomfort. On examination, tachycardia, elevated jugular venous pressure, paradoxical pulse, and narrow pulse pressure are seen. Kussmaul's sign is uncommon in cardiac tamponade. Diagnosis is confirmed by echocardiography and right-heart catheterization. Treatment involves intravascular fluid expansion and pericardiocentesis.

217-219. The answers are: 217-D, 218-B, 219-A. *(Hurst, ed 7. pp 158-160, 226-232.)* Tricuspid stenosis is characterized by a slow *y* descent of the jugular pulse and a diastolic rumble at the lower left sternal border.

Aortic regurgitation, in addition to generating the characteristic decrescendo diastolic murmur along the left sternal border, may also cause a diastolic rumble at the apex. Termed an Austin Flint murmur, this diastolic rumble is thought to result from the effect of the regurgitant jet of blood on the anterior leaflet of the mitral valve. Although distinguishing this murmur from that of mitral stenosis may be difficult, the absence of both an opening snap and loud first heart sound should suggest an Austin Flint murmur.

Constrictive pericarditis is characterized by a sharp *y* descent. This diagnosis should be considered in any patient who has unexplained edema or ascites.

220-223. The answers are: 220-D, 221-C, 222-A, 223-B. *(Braunwald, ed 3. pp 868-878. Hurst, ed 7. p 1173.)* Captopril, by inhibiting the angiotensin converting enzyme, is a potent antihypertensive agent because it prevents the generation of angiotensin II, a vasoconstrictor, and inhibits the degradation of bradykinin, a vasodilator. While especially useful in renovascular hypertension, it may cause membranous glomerulopathy, the nephrotic syndrome, and leukopenia.

Hydralazine is an arterial vasodilator generally used in conjunction with drugs that prevent reflex sympathetic stimulation of the heart, such as beta blockers and methyldopa. A lupus-like syndrome has been associated with the use of hydralazine.

Propranolol is a nonselective beta blocker and may therefore cause bronchospasm in susceptible patients. Beta blockers, as a class, may reduce HDL cholesterol and increase serum triglyceride levels.

Minoxidil is a more potent vasodilator than hydralazine but its use is limited by a high incidence of hirsutism. Marked fluid retention may also occur.

Gynecomastia is not a side effect of the drugs listed, although spironolactone, a potassium-sparing diuretic, and methyldopa, a centrally acting antiadrenergic agent, are two antihypertensives that may cause this problem.

224-227. The answers are: 224-E, 225-D, 226-B, 227-A. *(Braunwald, ed 3. pp 215-217. Hurst, ed 7. pp 288-289.)* Hypokalemia typically increases automaticity of myocardial fibers, resulting in ectopic beats or arrhythmias. Electrocardiography in hypokalemia reveals flattening of the T wave and prominent U waves.

Hyperkalemia decreases the rate of spontaneous diastolic depolarization in all pacemaker cells. It also results in slowing of conduction. One of the earliest electrocardiographic signs of hyperkalemia is the appearance of tall, peaked T waves. More severe elevations of the serum potassium result in widening of the QRS complex.

Hypocalcemia results in prolongation of the QT interval. Low serum calcium levels may also be associated with a decrease in myocardial contractility.

At serum sodium levels compatible with life, neither hyponatremia nor hypernatremia results in any characteristic electrocardiographic abnormalities.

228-230.   The answers are: 228-A, 229-D, 230-C. *(Braunwald, ed 3. pp 898, 1628-1629.)* Dextrocardia is a prominent feature of Kartagener's syndrome, an inherited condition that features situs inversus, chronic sinusitis, and bronchiectasis.

Dilatation of the aortic and pulmonary arteries commonly occurs with homocystinuria, an inborn error of metabolism. This condition, which is caused by a deficiency of the enzyme cystathionine synthetase, is characterized by the presence of intravascular thrombosis, lens subluxation, and osteoporosis, as well as large-vessel dilatation.

Hyperextensible joints, one of the common defects in Down's syndrome (trisomy 21), are frequently associated with cardiac abnormalities, including an endocardial cushion defect, atrial and ventricular septal defects, and the tetralogy of Fallot. Hypotonia often accompanies the hyperextensible joints.

231-235.   The answers are: 231-A, 232-D, 233-E, 234-B, 235-A. *(Braunwald, ed 3. pp 61-63. Hurst, ed 7. pp 157-160.)* The normal jugular venous pulse wave consists of three positive waves and two troughs. Normally, the a wave is the largest wave and is due to right atrial contraction. The c wave that follows is probably related to bulging of the tricuspid valve into the atrium. Relaxation of the atrium and downward displacement of the tricuspid valve toward the apex during ventricular systole result in the x descent. The v wave results from the filling of the right atrium with blood while the tricuspid valve is still closed. The y descent is the result of opening of the tricuspid valve and ventricular filling. An S_4 gallop is produced by atrial contraction and thus would occur at approximately the same time as the a wave.

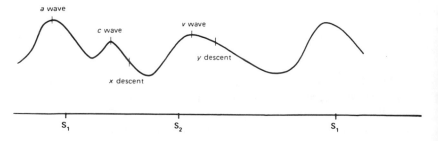

236-239.   The answers are: 236-C, 237-A, 238-D, 239-B. *(Braunwald, ed 3. pp 235-236, 1682-1684.)* Probability analysis is useful in clinical decision making. Frequently used terms are defined below. A true positive (TP) test is one that gives a positive result in a patient with disease. A true negative (TN) test is one that gives a negative result in a patient without disease. A false positive (FP) test is one that gives a positive result in a patient without disease. A false negative (FN) test is one that gives a negative result in a patient with disease.

The term *sensitivity* refers to the percentage of patients who will test positive out of all patients who have disease. The term *specificity* refers to the percentage of patients who will test negative out of all patients who are free of disease. The predictive value of a positive test refers to the percentage of true positives out of all positive tests. The predictive value of a negative test refers to the percentage of true negatives out of all negative tests. The sensitivity and specificity of a test cannot alone assess the probability of presence of disease. Bayes' theorem, which includes prevalence of disease in the population under study as well as the sensitivity and specificity of the testing method, is a useful tool in assessing the probability of presence of disease in an individual. For example, an exercise stress test demonstrating a 1-mm horizontal ST-segment depression is likely to represent a false positive test for ischemia in a 6-year-old girl and is likely to represent a true positive test for ischemia in a 60-year-old male smoker with hyperlipidemia and hypertension.

240-243.   The answers are: 240-D, 241-B, 242-C, 243-A. *(Braunwald, ed 3. pp 22-24. Hurst, ed 7. pp 154-157.)* Pulsus parvus et tardus is the small-amplitude pulse with slow rate of rise and delayed systolic peak that is characteristic of severe aortic stenosis.

Pulsus alternans is an alternation of the amplitude of the pulse that can be detected when systolic blood pressure varies by more than 20 mmHg from beat to beat. This is a sign of severe depression of myocardial function occurring during regular rhythm and can be confused with pulsus bigeminus, in which alternation of the pulse amplitude occurs as a result of bigeminal rhythm.

Pulsus paradoxus is a decrease in the amplitude of the arterial pulse during inspiration by greater than 10 mmHg and is palpable when an inspiratory drop in systolic pressure of greater than 20 mmHg occurs. Lesser degrees of pulsus paradoxus can be detected by sphygmomanometry and auscultation. Pulsus paradoxus is an exaggerated form of the normal inspiratory decrease in systolic pressure and is due to increased right ventricular stroke volume, decreased left ventricular stroke volume, and the effect of negative intrathoracic pressure on the aorta.

Pulsus bisferiens is a pulse with two systolic peaks that occurs in hypertrophic obstructive cardiomyopathy and in other conditions in which a large stroke volume is rapidly ejected from the left ventricle. In hypertrophic obstructive cardiomyopathy, rapid ejection of blood during early systole results in a prominent percussion wave, followed by a rapid decline in pulse as outflow obstruction occurs, and then followed by the tidal (reflected) wave. In hypertrophic obstructive cardio-myopathy, the magnitude of the bisferiens pulse is related to the degree of obstruction to left ventricular outflow. In patients with minor degrees of obstruction, the bisferiens pulse may be elicited by hemodynamic maneuvers such as Valsalva or inhalation of amyl nitrite.

Endocrinology and Metabolic Disease

DIRECTIONS: Each question below contains five suggested responses. Select the **one best** response to each question.

244. A 15½-year-old boy and his parents are concerned about the absence of any signs of puberty. His friends have all entered puberty and he feels embarrassed. He is nervous but well and his growth curves for height and weight are adequate. The physician asks the boy if his ability to smell is impaired. He thinks it is but as he did not volunteer the information his physician is uncertain of the significance of the answer. Physical examination is unrevealing except for prepubertal testes. His physician should consider all the following tests and recommendations EXCEPT

(A) basal serum levels of follicle-stimulating hormone (FSH), luteinizing hormone (LH), and testosterone
(B) serum prolactin
(C) a provocative test for growth hormone secretion, such as insulin tolerance test
(D) thyroid function tests
(E) evaluation of olfactory nerve function by smell testing

245. A 42-year-old woman is evaluated for hypoglycemia. She has experienced recurrent episodes of inappropriate behavior and dizziness for the past year, and she had syncope on one occasion after mowing her lawn. She denies hunger or palpitations and only occasionally has noted sweating. The patient has gained 15 pounds during the last year. Laboratory plasma studies reveal a glucose level of 65 mg/dL, insulin level of 18 μU/mL (normal: 10 to 20) after an overnight fast, and a diabetic glucose tolerance test (2-h value: 225 mg/dL) without reactive hypoglycemia. After 48 h of fasting, the patient became confused. At this time her plasma glucose and insulin levels are 34 mg/dL and 20 μU/mL, respectively. The most likely diagnosis is

(A) Addison's disease
(B) reactive hypoglycemia
(C) diabetes mellitus
(D) insulinoma
(E) hepatoma

246. The patient pictured below complains of the sudden onset of a painful "lump" in her neck following an upper respiratory infection. Physical examination reveals a soft, round, tender, midline mass at the level of the hyoid bone. The most likely diagnosis is

(A) acute suppurative thyroiditis
(B) subacute thyroiditis
(C) thyroglossal duct cyst
(D) toxic nodular goiter
(E) thyroid adenoma

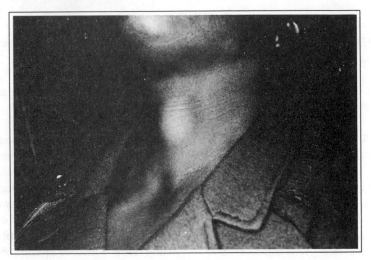

247. A 25-year-old woman who has insulin-dependent diabetes develops recurrent hypoglycemia. Her history reveals amenorrhea of 2 months' duration. A urinalysis is negative for glucose and protein; a vaginal smear shows no evidence of estrogen deficiency. The most likely diagnosis is

(A) pregnancy
(B) renal failure
(C) hypopituitarism
(D) insulinoma
(E) hyperthyroidism

248. A 25-year-old woman with a history of normal onset of menses is found on physical examination to have a blood pressure of 175/110 mmHg, clitoromegaly, and hirsutism. Laboratory values reveal a potassium of 3.0 and depressed aldosterone and plasma renin activity levels. The likely diagnosis for this patient is

(A) 11 β-hydroxylase deficiency
(B) 17 α-hydroxylase deficiency
(C) Addison's disease
(D) 21-hydroxylase deficiency
(E) none of the above

Endocrinology and Metabolic Disease 111

249. A 27-year-old woman presents with shortness of breath. Chest film reveals a bilateral pulmonary infiltrate. Her radiologic skeletal survey is negative. Laboratory serum values are as follows:

Chloride: 98 meq/L
Calcium: 11.9 mg/dL
(normal 9 to 11)
Phosphorus: 3.6 mg/dL
(normal 3 to 4.5)
Uric acid: 8.5 mg/dL
(normal 1.5 to 6.0)
Alkaline phosphatase: 50 U/L
(normal 21–91)

Blood urea nitrogen is 20 mg/dL. Pulmonary function tests reveal reduced vital capacity and reduced carbon monoxide diffusing capacity. Flat plate x-ray of the abdomen reveals bilateral nephrocalcinosis. The appropriate treatment for this patient is

(A) parathyroid exploration followed by subtotal parathyroidectomy
(B) potassium phosphate, 2 g daily
(C) mithramycin, 25 μg/kg body weight
(D) cyclophosphamide, 2 mg/kg daily
(E) prednisone, 50 mg daily

250. A patient develops severe hypotension immediately after removal of a pheochromocytoma. The most appropriate management would be the administration of which of the following?

(A) Corticosteroids
(B) Mineralocorticoids
(C) Alpha-stimulating agents
(D) Beta-stimulating agents
(E) Blood or plasma

251. A 30-year-old man is evaluated for a thyroid nodule. The patient reports that his father died from "thyroid cancer" and that a brother had a history of recurrent renal stones. Blood calcitonin concentration is 2000 pg/mL (normal: less than 100); serum calcium and phosphate levels are normal. Before referring the patient to a surgeon, the physician should

(A) obtain a liver scan
(B) perform a calcium infusion test
(C) measure urinary catecholamines
(D) administer suppressive doses of thyroxine and measure levels of thyroid-stimulating hormone
(E) treat the patient with radioactive iodine

252. A 32-year-old woman has a 3-year history of oligomenorrhea that has progressed to amenorrhea during the past year. She has observed loss of breast fullness, reduced hip measurements, acne, increased body hair, and deepening of her voice. Physical examination reveals frontal balding, clitoral hypertrophy, and a male escutcheon. Urinary free cortisol and dehydroepiandrosterone sulfate (DHEAS) are normal. Her plasma testosterone level is 6 ng/mL (normal: 0.2 to 0.8). The most likely diagnosis of this patient's disorder is

(A) hilar cell tumor
(B) Cushing's syndrome
(C) arrhenoblastoma
(D) polycystic ovary syndrome
(E) granulosa-theca cell tumor

253. An otherwise healthy 60-year-old man is noted on routine examination to have a firm thyroid nodule. Serum thyroxine is 8.0 μg/dL (normal: 4 to 11). Thyroid scan demonstrates a "cold" nodule. The most appropriate management would be which of the following procedures?

(A) Complete lobectomy
(B) Fine-needle aspiration cytology
(C) Levothyroxine
(D) Radioactive iodine therapy
(E) External irradiation

254. A 35-year-old woman has a 6-month history of amenorrhea. A 5-day course of medroxyprogesterone acetate (Provera), 10 mg, fails to induce withdrawal bleeding, while vaginal bleeding occurs following 20 days of conjugated estrogen (1.25 mg) administration. Her serum luteinizing and follicle-stimulating hormones are markedly increased. These findings are most consistent with which of the following abnormalities?

(A) Pituitary adenoma
(B) Polycystic ovary syndrome
(C) Endometrial failure
(D) Premature menopause
(E) Functional disorder

255. A 60-year-old woman presents with generalized muscle weakness, loss of appetite, palpitations, and a small diffuse nodular goiter. An electrocardiogram reveals rapid atrial fibrillation. Despite adequate digitalization, there is little slowing of her ventricular rate. Thyroid function studies reveal a serum thyroxine level of 12 μg/dL (normal: 5 to 12), with a triiodothyronine (T_3) level of 200 ng/dL (normal: 80 to 160), as measured by radioimmunoassay and a highly sensitive thyroid-stimulating hormone (TSH) of 0.05 μIU/mL (normal 0.3–3.0). The most likely diagnosis and appropriate treatment would be

(A) typical Graves' disease; therapy with antithyroid drugs
(B) mild Graves' disease; initiation of therapy with low dose of [131]I
(C) toxic multinodular goiter; therapy with antithyroid drugs followed by surgery
(D) toxic multinodular goiter; initiation of therapy with antithyroid agents followed by high dose of ^{131}I when euthyroid
(E) sick euthyroid syndrome; continuation of treatment of heart disease with digoxin and propranolol

256.   A 54-year-old man who has had a Billroth II procedure for peptic ulcer disease now presents with abdominal pain and is found to have recurrent ulcer disease. The physician is considering this patient's illness to be secondary either to a retained antrum or to a gastrinoma. Which of the following tests would best differentiate the two conditions?

(A) Random gastrin level
(B) Determination of 24-h acid production
(C) Serum calcium level
(D) Secretin infusion
(E) Insulin-induced hypoglycemia

257.   An active 24-year-old woman is found to have Hodgkin's disease on the basis of a cervical node biopsy. Chest x-ray reveals an anterior mediastinal mass, but lymphangiogram and liver biopsy are negative. Radiotherapy to the involved lymph nodes results in clinical remission; however, 2 months later the patient develops clinical and laboratory evidence of hypothyroidism. The most likely cause for hypothyroidism in this patient is

(A) Hashimoto's thyroiditis
(B) iodine deficiency
(C) iodine excess
(D) lymphomatous infiltration of the thyroid
(E) hypopituitarism

258.   A 55-year-old woman who has a history of severe depression and who had radical mastectomy for carcinoma of the breast 1 year previously develops polyuria, nocturia, and excessive thirst. Laboratory values are as follows:

Serum electrolytes (meq/L):
    Na^+ 149; K^+ 3.6
Serum calcium: 9.5 mg/dL
Blood glucose: 110 mg/dL
Blood urea nitrogen: 30 mg/dL
Urine osmolality: 150 mOsm/kg

The most likely diagnosis is

(A) psychogenic polydipsia
(B) renal glycosuria
(C) hypercalciuria
(D) diabetes insipidus
(E) inappropriate antidiuretic hormone syndrome

DIRECTIONS: Each question below contains four suggested responses of which **one or more** is correct. Select

A	if	**1, 2, and 3**	are correct
B	if	**1 and 3**	are correct
C	if	**2 and 4**	are correct
D	if	**4**	is correct
E	if	**1, 2, 3, and 4**	are correct

259. A 45-year-old man is noted on physical examination to have coarse facial features, oily skin, and an enlarged tongue. Initial laboratory studies reveal a fasting glucose of 190 mg/dL. Which of the following would support the physician's presumptive diagnosis of acromegaly?

(1) An increase in growth hormone with oral glucose administration
(2) Thyromegaly
(3) Signs consistent with carpal tunnel syndrome
(4) Normal basal growth hormone levels with elevated somatomedin C

260. Correct statements regarding the laboratory findings in patients who have Cushing's syndrome include which of the following?

(1) The presence of an abnormal diurnal steroid rhythm is diagnostic of the disorder
(2) An abnormal overnight dexamethasone suppression test (1 mg) is diagnostic of the disorder
(3) An exaggerated increase in plasma cortisol is usually observed following insulin-induced hypoglycemia
(4) Profound hypokalemia is suggestive of malignancy

261. A thin, 30-year-old woman complains of nervousness, mild sweating, palpitations, scanty menses, and weight loss. Her blood pressure is 150/80 mmHg and pulse rate 96 beats per minute. She displays mild hyperpigmentation and telangiectasis on the face. A small thyroid nodule is palpable. Serum thyroxine is 9.0 μg/dL (normal: 4.5 to 10); resin T_3 uptake is normal; radioactive iodine uptake is 30 percent (normal: 5 to 35); and thyroid scan shows uptake by a solitary left-sided thyroid nodule (no uptake by the right lobe). The diagnosis of hyperthyroidism in this patient may be established by

(1) thyrotropin-releasing hormone test
(2) serum triiodothyronine radioimmunoassay
(3) highly sensitive serum thyroid-stimulating hormone assay
(4) thyroid-stimulating immuno-globulin (TSI) assay

262. A 42-year-old man complains of impotence. His physician discovers that he is taking a drug that is known to interfere with the hormonal control of erection. Drugs having such an effect include

(1) chlorpheniramine
(2) spironolactone
(3) azathioprine
(4) cimetidine

263. Correct statements concerning the management of impending thyroid storm include that

(1) antithyroid drugs should be given prior to saturated solution of potassium iodine
(2) propranolol may help to control marked sinus tachycardia
(3) dexamethasone inhibits the generation of T_3 from T_4
(4) methimazole is as efficacious as propylthiouracil

264. A 20-year-old man who has a history of polyuria and hypotonic urine is placed on restricted water intake. After a period of dehydration his urine osmolality stabilizes at 450 mOsm/kg. Following injection of vasopressin (Pitressin) his urine osmolality rises to 600 mOsm/kg. This patient's symptoms are likely to improve if he is treated with

(1) chlorpropamide
(2) thiazide diuretics
(3) deamino-D-arginine vasopressin (dDAVP, desmopressin)
(4) glyburide

265. A 25-year-old woman complains of a recent onset of nervousness, palpitations, and increased sweating. Her serum thyroxine is 15 μg/dL (normal: 4 to 11), and radioactive iodine uptake is 1 percent. Hyperthyroidism in this patient may have been induced by

(1) thyroxine
(2) thyroiditis
(3) cholecystography
(4) oat cell carcinoma of the lungs

266. Correct statements about male infertility include which of the following?

(1) It can be associated with repeated respiratory tract infections
(2) A low plasma testosterone level necessitates a repeat measurement with simultaneous assessment of luteinizing hormone (LH) and follicle-stimulating hormone (FSH)
(3) Elevation of serum prolactin is more likely to be associated with a large rather than a small pituitary tumor
(4) Hypospermia is most likely caused by a readily detectable hormonal abnormality

267. Hyperparathyroidism with marked hypercalcemia is associated with which of the following abnormalities?

(1) Moniliasis
(2) Personality disturbances
(3) Prolonged QT interval on electrocardiogram
(4) Intense pruritus

268. A 30-year-old man complains of symptoms of sinusitis. Sinus x-rays incidentally show enlargement of the sella turcica. These findings are consistent with a diagnosis of

(1) pituitary adenoma
(2) craniopharyngioma
(3) empty-sella syndrome
(4) internal carotid artery aneurysm

SUMMARY OF DIRECTIONS

A	B	C	D	E
1, 2, 3	1, 3	2, 4	4	All are
only	only	only	only	correct

269. Cushing's syndrome is characterized by which of the following statements?

(1) The cause is most likely to be a pituitary microadenoma
(2) Although truncal obesity is generally present, a redistribution of weight is characteristic and approximately half the affected patients exhibit no weight gain
(3) Adrenal hyperplasia secondary to either pituitary or nonendocrine ACTH production can often be differentiated by a high-dosage dexamethasone suppression test
(4) The dexamethasone suppression test is less useful in screening for this syndrome than the now generally available radioimmunoassay for ACTH

270. Correct statements concerning subacute thyroiditis (de Quervain's thyroiditis) include which of the following?

(1) Pain, both localized and referred, is characteristic
(2) The erythrocyte sedimentation rate is increased and radioactive iodine uptake decreased
(3) The thyroid is extremely tender and occasionally nodular
(4) A transitory hyperthyroid phase is followed by hypothyroidism and recovery

271. Gynecomastia is associated with which of the following situations?

(1) Cirrhosis
(2) Digitalis administration
(3) Puberty
(4) Hyperthyroidism

272. After an initial 2 to 3 h of insulin treatment for diabetic ketoacidosis, there is most often a significant decline in blood level of

(1) glucose
(2) β-hydroxybutyrate
(3) free fatty acids
(4) acetoacetate

273. Correct statements concerning diabetic retinopathy include which of the following?

(1) Microaneurysms are the initial sign
(2) Proliferative retinopathy can be effectively controlled by photocoagulation
(3) Albuminuria caused by diabetic nephropathy is nearly always associated with retinopathy
(4) Hemorrhage into the vitreous usually indicates permanent loss of vision

274. Hyperaldosteronism is often associated with

(1) diuretic therapy
(2) Cushing's syndrome
(3) malignant hypertension
(4) licorice ingestion

275. Hypercalcemia in sarcoidosis is associated with

(1) seasonal changes in serum calcium
(2) improvement following corticosteroid therapy
(3) reduced parathormone concentration
(4) brown tumors

276. Toxic nodular goiter (Plummer's disease) is associated with

(1) exophthalmos
(2) thyroid acropathy
(3) thyroid dermopathy
(4) onycholysis

277. A 15-year-old boy, hospitalized for a fractured pelvis, is restricted to complete bed rest. Which of the following laboratory abnormalities may result?

(1) Glucose intolerance
(2) Hypercalcemia
(3) Absent diurnal steroid rhythm
(4) Hyperparathyroidism

278. Correct statements about thyroid antibodies include which of the following?

(1) They may be observed in 20 percent of elderly women
(2) They may be observed in patients with Graves' disease
(3) They are usually observed in Hashimoto's thyroiditis
(4) They are usually observed in subacute thyroiditis

279. Active patients afflicted with Paget's disease (osteitis deformans) generally demonstrate elevated levels of which of the following substances?

(1) Serum alkaline phosphatase
(2) Serum calcium
(3) Urine hydroxyproline
(4) Urine calcium

280. A 24-year-old woman complains of chronic fatigue. She tires easily and at times feels almost as if she is going to pass out, especially when she overexerts herself. She has lost about 10 pounds over the last 3 months because she does not "feel like eating." She was told she was suffering from multiple allergies because of the presence of allergic cells in her blood. At mid-afternoon her blood sugar was 62 mg/dL. Her blood pressure is 90/60 mmHg, pulse 90 beats per minute, weight 105 pounds, and height 64 inches. Which of the following clinical and laboratory information should be ascertained immediately?

(1) Blood pressure in supine and standing positions
(2) Careful inspection of the skin and oral cavity
(3) Screening cosyntropin stimulation test
(4) Glucose and insulin levels after 72-h fast

281. A 26-year-old woman consults her gynecologist for amenorrhea. She has been on oral contraceptives for 5 years but these were discontinued 6 months ago when she had a serious accident that required her to remain in traction in the hospital for 4 weeks. During this time she became extremely anxious and agitated and she was treated with haloperidol. The drug was gradually withdrawn but she had no further menstrual periods. Her amenorrhea is consistent with which of the following endocrinologic or radiologic findings?

(1) Serum prolactin 75 ng/mL; negative magnetic resonance imaging (MRI) of hypothalamus and pituitary gland
(2) Serum prolactin 300 ng/mL; 10-mm pituitary defect detected by coronal CT with contrast
(3) Suprasellar mass containing calcifications and a cystic compartment seen on MRI
(4) TSH 20 μU/mL (normal 0.3 to 3 μU/mL) with T$_4$ 1.0 μg/dL (normal 4 to 12 μg/dL)

282. A 22-year-old woman was referred by an orthopedic surgeon who treated her for a stress fracture of the femur. Which of the following aspects of the history and physical examination would be consistent with the development of osteoporosis?

(1) She experiences amenorrhea when she increases her jogging to greater than 60 miles a week
(2) She jogs and diets to keep her weight below 115 pounds, which is 90 percent of her ideal body weight
(3) She develops bloating, flatulence, and abdominal discomfort when she drinks milk or eats milk products
(4) She had childhood obesity and developed large bones

283. Osteoporosis has been associated with which of the following?

(1) Thyroxine treatment that suppresses TSH to zero
(2) Renal tubular acidosis
(3) Rheumatoid arthritis
(4) Polycystic ovarian syndrome

DIRECTIONS: Each group of questions below consists of lettered headings followed by a set of numbered items. For each numbered item select the **one** lettered heading with which it is **most** closely associated. Each lettered heading may be used **once, more than once, or not at all.**

Questions 284–287

For each case presentation below, select the most likely alteration in lipoprotein metabolism.

    (A) Familial lipoprotein lipase dysfunction
    (B) Low-density lipoprotein (LDL) receptor disorder
    (C) Inborn error of apolipoprotein E
    (D) Increased production of very-low-density lipoproteins (VLDL)
    (E) Increased transfer of apolipoprotein C from VLDL to high-density lipoproteins (HDL)

284. A 45-year-old diabetic patient complains of intermittent claudication. Physical examination reveals xanthomas of the palmar and digital creases and tuberoeruptive xanthomas of the elbows. Serum cholesterol and triglycerides are 320 and 280 mg/dL, respectively

285. A 12-year-old girl complains of acute abdominal pain. Physical examination reveals eruptive xanthomas, hepatosplenomegaly, and lipemia retinalis. Blood drawn on hospital admission looks like "cream of tomato soup" with serum cholesterol and triglycerides of 840 and 4000 mg/dL, respectively

286. A 32-year-old man has chest pain on exertion and a strong family history of coronary artery disease. Xanthomas are present on his Achilles tendon. Serum cholesterol and triglycerides are 380 and 150 mg/dL, respectively

287. A 72-year-old man who is an active jogger with a normal cardiac exercise stress test

Questions 288–291

For each case presentation below, select the most appropriate diagnosis. (Laboratory values appear in the table below.)

   (A) Adrenal carcinoma
   (B) Congenital adrenal hyperplasia
   (C) Cushing's disease
   (D) Oat cell carcinoma of the lung
   (E) Nelson's syndrome

288. A 45-year-old man complains of severe weakness. He appears chronically wasted and is mildly hyperpigmented. His blood pressure is 160/100 mmHg. A high-dose dexamethasone suppression test (2 mg every 6 h) causes no suppression of urinary free cortisol, 17-hydroxycorticosteroids (17-OHCS), or 17-ketosteroids (17-KS)

289. A 26-year-old woman complains of irregular menses, obesity, and low back pain. She has mild hypertension, central obesity, broad striae, acne, and mild hirsutism. A low-dose dexamethasone suppression test (0.5 mg every 6 h) causes no suppression of urinary free cortisol and 17-OHCS. A high-dose dexamethasone suppression test causes greater than 50 percent suppression of urinary free cortisol and 17-OHCS

290. A 20-year-old woman complains of weakness, easy bruising, hirsutism, and irregular menses. She exhibits a moon face, central obesity, and severe hirsutism involving the face and trunk, but no virilism. A high-dose dexamethasone suppression test causes no suppression of free cortisol, 17-OHCS, or 17-KS. Plasma dehydroepiandrosterone (DHEA) sulfate is fourfold normal

291. A 15-year-old boy complains of short stature. He has a history of early sexual development and accelerated growth that ceased 5 years ago. He displays hyperpigmentation. A high-dose dexamethasone suppression test causes greater than 50 percent suppression of urinary 17-KS

Laboratory Values					
Serum		Plasma		Urine	
K⁺	HCO₃	Cortisol at 8 A.M.	ACTH	17-OHCS	17-KS
Patient Number (meq/L)	(meq/L)	(μg/100 mL)*	(pg/100 mL)†	(mg/24h)★	(mg/24h)‡
288.	3.0	35	40	1000	35	40
289.	3.9	25	20	90	15	15
290.	3.2	32	80	5	35	70
291.	3.8	25	13	250	4	65

*Normal: 10 to 24.   ★Normal: 3 to 12.
†Normal: 40 to 100.   ‡Normal: 5 to 20.

DIRECTIONS: Each group of questions below consists of four lettered headings followed by a set of numbered items. For each numbered item select

A	if the item is associated with	(A) **only**
B	if the item is associated with	(B) **only**
C	if the item is associated with	**both** (A) and (B)
D	if the item is associated with	**neither** (A) nor (B)

Each lettered heading may be used **once, more than once, or not at all.**

Questions 292–296

(A) Multiple endocrine neoplasia, type I (MEN I)
(B) Multiple endocrine neoplasia, type II (MEN II)
(C) Both
(D) Neither

292. Medullary thyroid carcinoma

293. Multicentric parathyroid involvement

294. Increased ratio of urinary epinephrine to norepinephrine

295. Peptic ulcer disease is the major cause of morbidity and mortality

296. Carcinoid tumors

Questions 297–301

(A) Propylthiouracil (PTU)
(B) Methimazole
(C) Both
(D) Neither

297. Decrease in the peripheral conversion of T_4 to T_3

298. Inhibition of the incorporation of iodide into thyroglobulin

299. Leukopenia

300. Interference with the release of previously formed thyroid hormone

301. Intrathyroidal concentrations reflected by serum levels

Endocrinology and Metabolic Disease

Answers

244. The answer is C. *(Med Lett Drugs Ther 25:106, 1983. Wilson, ed 12. pp 1769-1773.)* A delay in the onset of puberty is much more common in boys than in girls and is usually a psychological hazard that can be handled with appropriate counseling. Genetic factors are important, and a history of delayed puberty in a father or an older brother would strongly suggest that no further investigations are needed. A physician would obviously look for signs of malnutrition from primary or secondary causes, such as a catabolic illness like regional ileitis. Such systemic illnesses can inhibit growth and consequently lead to delay in puberty. Since the patient appears to be well with normal weight and growth, systemic disorders as well as defects in growth hormone secretory dynamics are unlikely. Thus, provocative testing of growth hormone secretion is not indicated in this patient. Common endocrinopathies must then be excluded, such as hyperthyroidism, hypothyroidism, and prolactin-secreting pituitary adenomas. Measurement of the serum prolactin will detect the last, but levels will also be elevated in hypothyroidism and other central nervous system tumors such as craniopharyngioma, which interferes with normal hypothalamic inhibitory regulation of prolactin secretion. Elevation of prolactin from any cause will interfere with sexual function and must be pursued by pituitary imaging studies. In the absence of prolactin abnormalities, defects in the hypothalamic-pituitary-testicular axis—such as genetic errors in the testes and idiopathic gonadotropin deficiencies—must be excluded. Elevation of FSH and LH indicates a primary testicular disorder such as Klinefelter's syndrome. Low gonadotropins are consistent with normal physiologic delay in puberty but also with a defect in the hypothalamus or pituitary. The most common defect is a lack of hypothalamic secretion of luteinizing hormone releasing factor (LHRF). Such a defect can occur in association with other symptoms and signs such as anosmia, color blindness, and midline skeletal deformities that cluster together as Kallman's syndrome. Thus, defects in olfaction are strongly suggestive of the syndrome. Diagnosis is confirmed by testing with gonadorelin, a synthetic form of LHRF.

245. The answer is D. *(Felig, ed 2. pp 1184-1187. Wilson, ed 12. pp 1759-1765.)* The case history presented in the question is classic for insulinoma. The predominance of exercise-induced hypoglycemia and weight gain is characteristic of this disorder. Affected patients may have plasma insulin levels within normal limits after an overnight fast, but the ratio of serum insulin to serum glucose concentration is greater than 0.4. These patients frequently have glucose intolerance after glucose ingestion. The failure of insulin to fall when fasting hypoglycemia develops establishes the diagnosis of hyperinsulinism. In contrast, patients having reactive hypoglycemia do not develop hypoglycemia with fasting. Although hepatoma and Addison's disease may be associated with fasting hypoglycemia, insulin values fall appropriately during a fast in these disorders.

246. The answer is C. *(Wilson, ed 12. pp 1709–1712.)* Thyroglossal duct cyst is the most important anomaly of thyroid development. Excision of the cyst is generally indicated because of the cyst's propensity for infection. Infection may enter the duct if a communication persists with the pharynx through the foramen cecum at the base of the tongue. After an acute upper respiratory infection, the duct may become obstructed. The obstruction can lead to cystic dilatation, thereby making the lesion clinically apparent.

247. The answer is A. *(Felig, ed 2. pp 1155–1162. Wilson, ed 12. p 1785.)* Insulin-dependent diabetic women who desire pregnancy are advised to normalize their glucose control with frequent home glucose monitoring and multiple insulin injections prior to conception. This itself increases the risk of hypoglycemia. When pregnancy occurs, the risk is greater because of fetal utilization of glucose and gluconeogenic substrates. Later in pregnancy, insulin resistance occurs secondary to a rise in placental contrainsular hormones. In the patient presented in the question, diabetic nephropathy is highly unlikely because of the absence of proteinuria. Evidence of estrogen effect on vaginal smear makes hypopituitarism unlikely. Hyperthyroidism causes oligomenorrhea and generally produces an insulin-resistant state.

248. The answer is A. *(Wilson, ed 12. pp 1727–1728.)* Congenital adrenal hyperplasia is characterized by an inherited enzymatic defect of steroidogenesis that interferes with the normal feedback inhibition of ACTH secretion, thus resulting in adrenal hyperplasia; it is an autosomal recessive disorder. Of the various enzyme deficiencies, only two, 11 β-hydroxylase and 17 α-hydroxylase deficiencies, are associated with hypertension. In 11 β-hydroxylase deficiency, the block creates a deficiency of cortisol, corticosterone, and aldosterone. The resultant accumulation of deoxycorticosterone protects against adrenal insufficiency and leads to salt and water retention, and the consequent volume expansion causes a suppression of renin activity. While men are only affected by hypertension, women also experience some degree of virilization from excess androgen production. The condition is treated with small doses of dexamethasone to suppress ACTH and reduce deoxycorticosterone levels.

249. The answer is E. *(Felig, ed 2. pp 1415–1416.)* The clinical presentation of a bilateral pulmonary infiltrate, together with nephrocalcinosis, hypercalcemia, hyperuricemia, and normal phosphate levels, is typical of sarcoidosis. The absence of any bone lesion, together with a normal phosphate level, makes primary hyperparathyroidism unlikely. Furthermore, in primary hyperparathyroidism the serum chloride is frequently elevated and pulmonary infiltation, together with reduced vital capacity and diffusion defect, is uncharacteristic. The other causes of hypercalcemia are not associated with this clinical and biochemical constellation. The mechanism of hypercalcemia in sarcoidosis is related to hydroxylation of vitamin D by the giant cells of the granulomatous inflammation. 25-Hydroxyvitamin D_3 is further hydroxylated by the kidney to form 1,25-dihydroxyvitamin D_3, which stimulates calcium absorption in the intestine. Glucocorticoids inhibit formation of active vitamin D. To induce a remission, sarcoidosis is treated with prednisone, approximately 1 mg/kg per day.

250. The answer is E. *(Felig, ed 2. pp 667–672. Wilson, ed 12. pp 1735–1739.)* Patients who have pheochromocytoma frequently demonstrate reduced circulating plasma volume, probably as a consequence of chronic, excessive alpha-adrenergic stimulation. Reduced plasma volume is suggested clinically by orthostatic hypotension or by elevated hematocrit. If plasma volume is reduced preoperatively and not corrected by treatment with phenoxybenzamine and administration of copious amounts of fluid, severe hypotension may occur during surgery immediately after removal of the tumor. Hypotension under such circumstances is best treated with volume expansion (e.g., blood replacement) rather than with a vasoconstrictive agent.

251. The answer is C. *(Felig, ed 2. pp 1670–1675. Wilson, ed 12. pp 1811–1812.)* For the patient described in the question, the markedly increased calcitonin levels indicate the diagnosis of medullary carcinoma of the thyroid. In view of the family history, the patient most likely has multiple endocrine neoplasia (MEN) type II, which includes medullary carcinoma of the thyroid gland, pheochromocytoma, and parathyroid hyperplasia. Pheochromocytoma may exist without sustained hypertension as indicated by excessive urinary catecholamines. Before thyroid surgery is performed on this patient, a pheochromocytoma must be ruled out through urinary catecholamine determinations; the presence of such a tumor might expose him to a hypertensive crisis during surgery. The entire thyroid gland must be removed because foci of parafollicular cell hyperplasia, a premalignant lesion, may be scattered throughout the gland. Successful removal of the medullary carcinoma can be monitored with serum calcitonin levels. Hyperparathyroidism, while unlikely in this patient, is probably present in his brother.

252. The answer is C. *(Felig, ed 2. pp 964–966. Wilson, ed 12. pp 1727–1729.)* The symptoms of masculination (e.g., alopecia, deepening of voice, clitoral hypertrophy) in the patient presented in the question are characteristic of active androgen-producing tumors. Such extreme virilization is very rarely observed in polycystic ovary syndrome or in Cushing's syndrome; moreover, the presence of normal cortisol and markedly elevated plasma testosterone levels indicates an ovarian rather than adrenal cause of her findings. Although hilar cell tumors are capable of producing the picture seen in this patient, they are very rare and usually arise in postmenopausal women. Arrhenoblastomas are the most common androgen-producing ovarian tumors. Their incidence is highest during the reproductive years. Composed of varying proportions of Leydig's and Sertoli's cells, they are generally benign. In contrast to arrhenoblastomas, granulosa-theca cell tumors produce feminization, not virilization.

253. The answer is B. *(Wilson, ed 12. pp 1709–1711.)* The most serious diagnostic possibilities—i.e., anaplastic tumor, lymphoma or metastatic disease—will either be readily confirmed or highly suspected by thyroid cytology. The more indolent tumors such as papillary or follicular carcinomas may also be diagnosed if the specimen is highly cellular or there are neoplastic features in the cytology. Otherwise a benign cytology would permit a cautious trial of exogenous levothyroxine suppression to determine if the nodule regresses in size over 6 to 12 months. Radioactive iodine therapy and external irradiation are used to treat thyroid carcinoma postoperatively.

254. The answer is D. *(Felig, ed 2. pp 977–980. Wilson, ed 12. pp 1783–1789.)* The failure of the patient presented in the question to respond to medroxyprogesterone acetate (Provera) indicates estrogen deficiency, while her ability to respond to estrogens rules out endometrial failure (e.g., Asherman's syndrome) as a basis for her disorder. Since patients who have polycystic ovary syndromes continue to produce estrogens, they would be expected to exhibit both withdrawal bleeding after Provera and relatively normal production of gonadotropins. In the patient under discussion, a diagnosis of ovarian failure or premature menopause is indicated by the marked increase in gonadotropins. In contrast, patients suffering from pituitary tumors and functional disorders have reduced gonadotropins.

255. The answer is D. *(Wilson, ed 12. pp 1702–1706.)* The clinical description is typical of apathetic hyperthyroidism, which may be caused by subtle Graves' disease or toxic multinodular goiter. The signs of hyperthyroidism are attenuated in the later decades of life and women are affected much more frequently than men. The clinical presentation differs from that of Graves' disease because of the absence of exophthalmos. Thyrotoxic cardiac disease is extremely common. Goiter may not be palpable. Resistance to the usual therapeutic dosages of digitalis is common. The syndrome of sick euthyroidism is more commonly associated with low serum thyroxine and triiodothyronine values in debilitated elderly patients. The treatment of choice for this patient is radioactive iodine, and large doses, usually in excess of 20 μCi/g of estimated thyroid mass, are required. In order to prevent an exacerbation of thyrotoxic symptoms caused by the destruction of the thyroid gland and the release of thyroxine as a result of a radiation-induced thyroiditis, it is prudent to initiate therapy with antithyroid agents and administer the radioactive iodine as a definitive treatment only when the affected patient has become euthyroid.

256. The answer is D. *(Wilson, ed 12. pp 1239-1243, 1811.)* The diagnosis of gastrinoma should be considered in all patients with either recurrent ulcers after surgical correction for peptic ulcer disease, ulcers in the distal duodenum or jejunum, ulcer disease associated with diarrhea, or evidence suggestive of the multiple endocrine neoplasia (MEN) type I (familial association of pituitary, para-thyroid, and pancreatic tumors) in ulcer patients. Because basal serum gastrin and basal acid production may both be normal or only slightly elevated in patients with gastrinomas, provocative tests may need to be employed for diagnosis. Both the secretin and calcium infusion tests are used; a paradoxical increase in serum gastrin concentration is seen in response to both infusions in patients with gastrinomas. In contrast, other conditions associated with hypergastrinemia such as duodenal ulcers, retained antrum, gastric outlet obstruction, antral G-cell hyperplasia, and pernicious anemia will respond with either no change or a decrease in serum gastrin.

257. The answer is C. *(Felig, ed 2. pp 76-77, 417. Wilson, ed 12. p 1694.)* The patient presented in the question has a classic case of iodine-induced hypothy-roidism (Wolff-Chaikoff effect). Normally, patients rapidly escape the suppressive effects of iodine on thyroid hormone production so that circulating thyroid hor-mone levels are unaffected. However, patients who are exposed to neck radiation (external or radioactive iodine) or who have glandular damage (thyroiditis or Graves' disease) are at risk of hypothyroidism. The source of iodine in this patient is the lymphangiogram, a procedure that would be expected to increase the patient's iodine pool for several years. Hypothyroidism occurring many years after external radiation is not uncommon in patients who have been treated for head, neck, and mediastinal tumors.

258. The answer is D. *(Felig, ed 2. pp 357-368. Wilson, ed 12. pp 1684-1689.)* Metastatic tumors rarely cause diabetes insipidus but of the tumors that may cause it, carcinoma of the breast is by far the most common. In the patient dis-cussed in the question, the diagnosis of diabetes insipidus is suggested by hyper-natremia and a low urine osmolality. Psychogenic polydipsia is an unlikely diag-nosis since serum sodium is usually mildly reduced in this condition. Renal glycosuria would be expected to induce a higher urine osmolality than this patient has because of the osmotic effect of glucose. While nephrocalcinosis secondary to hypercalcemia may produce polyuria, hypercalciuria does not. Finally, the findings of inappropriate antidiuretic hormone syndrome are the opposite of those observed in diabetes insipidus and thus incompatible with the clinical picture in this patient.

259.   The answer is E (all). *(Wilson, ed 12. pp 1660-1664.)* Hypersecretion of growth hormone is usually secondary to a somatotropic pituitary cell adenoma. Prior to epiphyseal closure, an increase in growth rate with minimal bony deformity is the common presentation; in adults, coarsening of facial features, soft tissue swelling of hands and feet, and bony proliferation are typical manifestations. Diagnosis rests on characteristics of growth hormone secretion that are unique to acromegalics. Random serum determinations range from normal to grossly elevated but an oral glucose tolerance test fails to suppress serum growth hormone levels. In contrast, 70 to 80 percent of patients with acromegaly actually increase growth hormone in response to glucose. Acromegaly may be caused by micropituitary tumors (less than 10 mm) that maintain normal growth hormone levels, but the absence of physiologic regulation causes increased levels of somatomedin C produced in the liver in response to growth hormone. Thyromegaly, frequently seen in acromegaly, is indicative of growth hormone's effect in stimulating generalized organomegaly. Similarly, carpal tunnel syndrome indicates bony overgrowth.

260.   The answer is D (4). *(Wilson, ed 12. pp 1720-1723.)* While an abnormal diurnal steroid rhythm is a hallmark of Cushing's syndrome, it is a nonspecific finding and also may be observed in stress, obesity, or depression. Similarly, the overnight dexamethasone suppression test, virtually always abnormal in Cushing's syndrome, also may be abnormal in obesity, depression, severe illness, or in association with phenytoin (Dilantin) administration. Patients with Cushing's syndrome, in contrast to normal subjects, characteristically do not show an increase in blood cortisol after insulin-induced hypoglycemia. Profound hypokalemia indicates markedly elevated levels of cortisol, which are more likely found in patients with adrenal carcinoma or ectopic production of adrenocorticotropic hormone (ACTH).

261.   The answer is A (1, 2, 3). *(Felig, ed 2. p 418. Wilson, ed 12. pp 1702-1705.)* The clinical and laboratory findings in the patient presented in the question are most consistent with "T₃ toxicosis." This hyperthyroid state is a result of overproduction of triiodothyronine in the presence of normal or slightly elevated thyroxine. Radioactive iodine uptake may be normal or increased. "T₃ toxicosis" is observed most commonly in patients who have autonomous nodules or who have been treated for Graves' disease. The diagnosis is established either by the presence of elevated serum triiodothyronine (radioimmunoassay) or suppression of the highly sensitive thyroid-stimulating hormone (HS-TSH) assay. If HS-TSH assay is not available, then the failure to stimulate TSH release by injection of thyrotropin-releasing hormone is consistent with hyperthyroidism. In the patient presented, serum thyroid-stimulating immunoglobulin (TSI) would not be present. TSI is observed in Graves' disease but not in the presence of an autonomous nodule.

2;62.   The answer is C (2, 4). *(Spark, JAMA 243:750, 1980. Wilson, ed 12. pp 296-299.)* Although psychological causes of impotence are responsible for the majority of cases, there are many drugs that have impotence as a side effect. Diuretics, methyldopa, clonidine, and beta blockers can produce complete or incomplete impotence. Recently it has been discovered that the widely used drugs cimetidine and spironolactone act as antiandrogens; in antagonizing the effects of androgen on the target tissue, they can affect the hormonal control of erection. While it is important to stress that the majority of patients taking these drugs do not suffer from impotence, physicians need to be aware of this possibility as these drugs have not been traditionally thought of in this context. Although clinical skills remain the best tools for sorting out the different causes of impotence, there are disturbances in endocrine function that may be responsible. Usually the measurement of plasma testosterone and prolactin in patients who have been consistently impotent for a period of more than 3 months will allow physicians to decide which patients have abnormalities of the endocrine system that require a more detailed evaluation. In one recent study of 105 patients presenting with impotence, 37 were found to have organic hypogonadism. Twenty of these patients had a hypothalamic pituitary deficiency. The incidence of impotence associated with antihypertensive treatment is as high as 17 percent.

263.   The answer is A (1, 2, 3). *(Wilson, ed 12. pp 1708–1709.)* Thyroid storm is an acute exacerbation of partially treated or untreated thyrotoxicosis evoked by a precipitating factor such as infection, trauma, surgery, diabetic ketoacidosis, or pregnancy. The patient usually presents with fever, restlessness, nausea and vomiting, abdominal pain, tachycardia, diaphoresis, and, rarely, delirium. Treatment involves antagonizing all facets of thyroid hormone synthesis. Propylthiouracil, because it inhibits the iodination of tyrosine and monoiodotyrosine and prevents the coupling of iodotyrosines to form T_3 and T_4, is a first-line agent in the treatment of storm. As it also prevents the conversion of T_4 to T_3, it is preferred over methimazole, which does not affect this final step. Once iodination is inhibited, large doses of iodine are then administered in order to prevent the release of thyroid hormones. Dexamethasone, in addition to assuring adequate glucocorticoid stores, supports the actions of both propylthiouracil and iodine by inhibiting glandular release of hormone and preventing the conversion of T_4 to T_3. Propranolol is also given in order to reduce the effects of the increased sympathetic state.

264.   The answer is A (1, 2, 3). *(Felig, ed 2. pp 357–368. Wilson, ed 12. pp 1684–1688.)* The ability of the patient presented in the question to concentrate urine clearly is impaired. His response to vasopressin (Pitressin) establishes the diagnosis of partial diabetes insipidus, thus ruling out psychogenic or nephrogenic causes for his urinary findings. Patients who have some antidiuretic hormone (ADH) secretion generally respond to chlorpropamide, thiazide diuretics, or dDAVP. Chlorpropamide enhances the action of ADH in the kidney. The negative salt balance induced by the diuretic leads to a reduction in glomerular filtration rate and to enhanced proximal tubular water reabsorption. This results in the delivery of less water to water-impermeable distal segments and so to reduced water excretion. dDAVP is a potent analogue of ADH. In contrast to chlorpropamide, the second-generation sulfonylureas glyburide and glipizide have no ADH-like effects.

265. The answer is A (1, 2, 3). *(Wilson, ed 12. p 1708.)* Thyrotoxicosis associated with decreased radioactive iodine (RAI) uptake has been observed in (1) patients who are surreptitiously taking thyroxine; (2) Graves' disease with iodine loading; (3) iodine-induced thyrotoxicosis (jodbasedow phenomenon); (4) acute phase of thyroiditis; (5) struma ovarii; and (6) metastatic follicular carcinoma. While a few rare cases of pituitary adenomas that produce thyroid-stimulating hormone (TSH) have been reported, in this condition RAI uptake would be increased. Oat cell carcinoma is associated with several ectopic hormone syndromes, including ectopic ACTH production and the syndrome of inappropriate antidiuretic hormone, but not with thyroid overproduction.

266. The answer is A (1, 2, 3). *(Wilson, ed 12. pp 1657-1660.)* Testicular function consists of two interrelated systems: one designed to produce sperm in spermatogenic tubules and the other to produce androgenic steroids. Testosterone is the most important androgen made in Leydig cells that are dispersed among the tubules. The major hormone regulating testosterone production is luteinizing hormone; follicle-stimulating hormone plays a less important role in the production of testosterone, but it is the major hormone regulating spermatogenesis. Male infertility can be associated with defects in both systems. Two syndromes have been identified that affect the cilia of the sperm, thus reducing their mobility and causing infertility. In Kartagener's syndrome the infertility is associated with situs inversus and the development of severe bronchiectasis. There is a defect in the protein dynein that is essential for the movement of both respiratory cilia and the sperm tail. In a second syndrome, this protein is normal but the radial spokes in the cilia are abnormal. Leydig cell function is assessed by obtaining plasma testosterone levels and, if they are low, exploring a pituitary cause for this defect by the simultaneous assay of plasma luteinizing hormone levels. Hyperprolactinemia is the most common cause of secondary hypogonadism. Because male sexuality is not inhibited by small decrements of LH and testosterone caused by prolactin-secreting pituitary tumors, these tumors are significantly enlarged at the onset of symptoms. Hypospermia is the most common abnormality causing male infertility and its cause in the majority of patients is not detectable.

267. The answer is C (2, 4). *(Felig, ed 2. pp 1379-1381. Wilson, ed 12. pp 1902-1906.)* Severe hyperparathyroidism is frequently associated with personality changes, ranging from lethargy and mild affective disorders to mental obtundation and psychosis. Pruritus, which may be intense in hyperparathyroidism, disappears following parathyroidectomy. The intensity of symptoms is related to the magnitude of the hypercalcemia. Most cases of hyperparathyroidism are currently being detected by finding mild hypercalcemia (less than 11.5 mg/dL) on serum multianalysis. These patients are asymptomatic and have either a subclinical disorder without other abnormalities or a subtle form of hyperparathyroidism confirmed by demonstrating elevated parathyroid hormone levels or increased phosphate excretion. Electrocardiographic changes generally are limited to a shortening of the QT interval. Moniliasis is associated with hypoparathyroidism, not hyperparathyroidism.

268. The answer is E (all). *(Wilson, ed 12. pp 1675-1678.)* Enlargement of the sella turcica is characteristic, but not diagnostic, of pituitary tumors. Suprasellar lesions like craniopharyngiomas and aneurysms may extend into the sella, producing enlargement of the sella and erosion of its walls. In addition, cerebrospinal fluid pressure can force the subarachnoid space into the sella, resulting in enlargement of the sella and compression of the normal pituitary (empty-sella syndrome). The differential diagnosis can be readily made by cross-sectional imaging of the hypothalamus and pituitary by computed tomography (CT) with contrast injection or magnetic resonance imaging (MRI) with gadolinium enhancement.

269. The answer is B (1, 3). *(Felig, ed 2. p 608. Wilson, ed 12. pp 1720-1723.)* Regardless of pathogenesis, Cushing's syndrome is characterized by excess production of cortisol. Most cases are due to bilateral adrenal hyperplasia secondary to overproduction of ACTH by a pituitary microadenoma. Harvey Cushing originally suggested (1932) that the excess ACTH was produced by pituitary basophil adenomas, a condition that was designated Cushing's disease before it was recognized that pituitary basophilism was only one of the causes of the syndrome that would bear his name. Tumors may be very small and difficult to detect or not present at all. Petrosal sinus vein catheterization for ACTH levels is being more commonly used to localize these microtumors. The 48-h dexamethasone suppression test is still an important screening test, since the failure of suppression of urinary 17-hydroxysteroid levels to less than 3 mg/24 h or of plasma cortisol levels to less than 5 μg/dL by this test is virtually diagnostic of the syndrome. The most common nonendocrine tumor that secretes ACTH is a small cell (oat cell) carcinoma of the lung. Some carcinoid tumors also produce ACTH but because of their indolent, slowly progressive course, they are difficult to discriminate from ACTH-producing pituitary microtumors. In these patients or in others with adrenal neoplasms, no suppression occurs after dexamethasone administration, since pituitary ACTH secretion is already suppressed by the elevated cortisol levels. While routine laboratory examinations are rarely of major diagnostic utility in the diagnosis of Cushing's syndrome, certain abnormalities are suggestive: high normal values of hemoglobin, hematocrit, and red-cell count; a total lymphocyte count below normal in 35 percent of patients, and an eosinophil count usually below 100/mm^3; and fasting hyperglycemia in 10 to 15 percent of patients.

270.   The answer is E (all). *(Wilson, ed 12. pp 1711-1712.)* Subacute thyroiditis is characterized by acute or subacute onset of asthenia, malaise, and pain over the thyroid that often is referred to the ear, lower jaw, or occiput. The disease is probably viral in origin; it frequently follows an upper respiratory infection. Subacute thyroiditis is diagnosed on the basis of an elevated erythrocyte sedimentation rate and a markedly depressed radioactive iodine uptake. Frequently, a high serum T_4 level is observed, which quickly drops to hypothyroid levels followed by a recovery phase.

271.   The answer is E (all). *(Felig, ed 2. pp 886-889. Wilson, ed 12. pp 1796-1798.)* Cirrhosis and uremia are among the most common causes of gynecomastia. Estrogen- and gonadotropin-secreting tumors and hypogonadism must also be considered as causes. In addition, exogenous estrogens, spironolactone, and digitalis may produce this abnormality. Gynecomastia occurs commonly during puberty, occasionally in association with hyperthyroidism, and after recovery from severe malnutrition.

272.   The answer is A (1, 2, 3). *(Wilson, ed 12. pp 1749-1752.)* Acetoacetate levels—in contrast to glucose, β-hydroxybutyrate, and free fatty acid levels—may actually rise during the first few hours of insulin treatment for diabetic ketoacidosis. Treatment decreases the $NADH^+/NAD$ ratio so that β-hydroxybutyrate, the major blood ketone, is converted to acetoacetate. Since testing material measures acetoacetate rather than β-hydroxybutyrate, serial measurements of serum ketones may show an increase or steady state reflecting the conversion to acetoacetate. However, total blood ketones, as measured by quantitative enzymatic techniques, may decline by 50 percent during the first few hours of treatment without a demonstrable change in serum ketones, as measured by Acetest tablets and Ketostix.

273.   The answer is A (1, 2, 3). *(Wilson, ed 12. pp 1753-1754.)* The earliest sign of retinal change in diabetes is increased permeability followed by occlusion of retinal capillaries with sacular and fusiform aneurysms. Proliferative retinopathy, also known as *neovascularization* because of growth of new blood vessels, is effectively treated by photocoagulation. This procedure reduces the risk of hemorrhage into the vitreous. The hemorrhage may be reabsorbed spontaneously or may require vitrectomy, which restores vision in over half of the patients. Retinopathy often occurs without albuminuria, the first sign of diabetic nephropathy. However, albuminuria without diabetic retinopathy is atypical of diabetic nephropathy and suggests another etiology.

274.   The answer is B (1, 3). *(Felig, ed 2. pp 751-764. Wilson, ed 12. pp 1716, 1725-1727.)* Diuretic therapy and malignant hypertension often induce excessive secretion of renin leading to secondary hyperaldosteronism, a condition that may be distinguished from primary hyperaldosteronism by elevated levels of renin. Renin is characteristically suppressed in primary hyperaldosteronism. Aldosterone levels are normal or low in Cushing's syndrome; hypokalemia in this disorder results from excessive cortisol and deoxycorticosterone production. Excessive licorice ingestion may produce hypokalemia and hypertension because of glycyrrhizic acid in the licorice. This mineralocorticoid-like substance expands plasma volume and reduces aldosterone secretion.

275. The answer is A (1, 2, 3). *(Felig, ed 2. pp 1415-1416. Wilson, ed 12. pp 1908-1909.)* The association of hypercalcemia with sarcoidosis is often most striking in summer and, in fact, may disappear in winter. This fluctuation probably is mediated by the effects of sunlight on vitamin D synthesis in skin. Characteristically, patients who have sarcoidosis, vitamin D intoxication, or certain malignancies demonstrate a fall in serum calcium after prednisone treatment (40 to 80 mg/day). Parathormone levels in hypercalcemic disorders not associated with hyperparathyroidism characteristically are low. Brown tumors are associated with hyperparathyroidism and represent areas of increased osteoclastic activity; they are not observed in sarcoidosis.

276. The answer is D (4). *(Felig, ed 2. pp 422-423. Wilson, ed 12. pp 1703-1707.)* Onycholysis, or distal separation of the nail bed, is observed in over 10 percent of patients who have hyperthyroidism resulting from either Graves' disease or toxic nodular goiter; it usually begins in the nail of the fourth finger. In contrast, thyroid dermopathy (formerly called pretibial myxedema) and exophthalmos are virtually pathognomonic of Graves' disease and are not observed in patients who have toxic nodular goiter. Thyroid acropathy, almost always associated with a history of exophthalmos and Graves' disease, is characterized by clubbing of the fingers and toes, swelling of the subcutaneous tissues of the extremities, and subperiosteal bone changes without new bone formation.

277. The answer is A (1, 2, 3). *(Felig, ed 2. pp 1416-1417. Wilson, ed 12. pp 1715, 1909.)* Patients who are restricted to total bed rest or subject to stress will demonstrate glucose intolerance that is a consequence of insulin resistance. Furthermore, immobilization of young patients undergoing rapid bone growth can result in hypercalcemia and hypercalciuria. The hypercalcemia, in turn, will suppress parathyroid secretion. The severe pain and stress of a fracture, such as in the boy presented in the question, could lead to the loss of normal diurnal rhythm for cortisol secretion.

278. The answer is A (1, 2, 3). *(Wilson, ed 12. pp 1698, 1712.)* More than 95 percent of patients who have Hashimoto's thyroiditis demonstrate high titers of thyroglobulin antibodies, thyroid microsomal antibodies, or both. Extremely high titers are virtually diagnostic of the disease. Lower titers of thyroid antibodies may be observed in 20 percent of elderly women and in patients with Graves' disease and other autoimmune diseases (e.g., pernicious anemia), as well as relatives of patients with Hashimoto's thyroiditis and Graves' disease.

279. The answer is B (1, 3). *(Felig, ed 2. pp 1483–1491. Wilson, ed 12. pp 1938–1941.)* Paget's disease is characterized by excessive and abnormal remodeling of bone. The markedly increased bone turnover leads to elevations in serum alkaline phosphatase level and in urine hydroxyproline excretion. Serum and urinary calcium levels are normal; however, during periods of immobilization, patients afflicted with Paget's disease can develop severe hypercalcemia and hypercalciuria.

280. The answer is A (1, 2, 3). *(Wilson, ed 12. pp 1729–1732.)* The patient has nonspecific symptoms consistent with the diagnosis of primary adrenal insufficiency, or Addison's disease. In contrast to patients with weakness secondary to functional causes, this patient has weight loss, eosinophilia, and low blood glucose and blood pressure. Orthostatic hypotension is found in 50 percent of the patients with Addison's disease. Evidence of subtle hyperpigmentation in the creases of the hand, the rough surface of the knees and elbows, or the mucosal membranes, such as gingiva or vagina, is found in 95 percent of the cases. Since Addison's disease can quickly decompensate into acute adrenal crisis, a cosyntropin test should be done as soon as possible. A normal response to this synthetic ACTH derivative is an increment in serum cortisol of at least 7 μg/dL, and a peak value over 18 μg/dL. This would exclude further consideration of the diagnosis. When the index of suspicion is high, patients are treated with glucocorticoid pending the test results. The 72-h fast is ordered to confirm the diagnosis of fasting hypoglycemia, which is usually caused by an insulinoma.

281. The answer is E (all). *(Wilson, ed 12. pp 1657–1660, 1675–1677.)* Serum prolactin is an essential test in her evaluation since hyperprolactinemia of any cause is associated with amenorrhea. Causes of hyperprolactinemia include prolactin-secreting pituitary microadenomas (usually defined as less than 10 mm diameter with serum prolactin less than 200 ng/mL) or macroadenomas; hypothalamic or pituitary disorders, such as tumors or sarcoidosis, which interfere with hypothalamic secretion of prolactin inhibitory factor; and functional disorders, including hypothyroidism and idiopathic hyperprolactinemia. Since changes in serum prolactin in response to stimulatory or inhibitory agents will not consistently differentiate a functional from an anatomic etiology for hyperprolactinemia, the diagnosis of functional hyperprolactinemia is made by exclusion of anatomic processes using MRI or CT. Thus, this patient may have functional hyperprolactinemia caused by estrogen's direct stimulatory effect on prolactin secretion, but this diagnosis can only be made following a negative MRI (choice 1). She may have a prolactin-secreting macroadenoma (choice 2) or a craniopharyngioma (choice 3), both of which are easily detected by CT or MRI. Hypothyroidism (choice 4) should always be excluded and treated prior to directly treating the hyperprolactinemia with bromo-criptine or other dopamine agonists.

282. The answer is A (1, 2, 3). *(Wilson, ed 12. pp 1921–1926.)* Intensive exercise does not protect women from developing osteoporosis if the exercise results in amenorrhea. Cyclic release of estrogens during a normal menstrual cycle, as well as adequate protein and mineral intake, is necessary for bones to develop normally and mature. Women who excessively exercise or assiduously maintain lean weights associated with amenorrhea are at risk of fractures from osteoporosis. Another risk factor for osteoporosis is reduced dietary calcium intake secondary to lactase defi-ciency or alcoholism. In contrast, women with early onset of obesity develop a large bone frame, which is considered to be secondary to increased nutrient intake and protects them to some extent from osteoporosis.

283. The answer is B (1, 3). *(Wilson, ed 12. pp 1922–1930.)* Osteoporosis is a complication of many systemic disorders. Hyperthyroidism increases calcium turn-over of bone, which can result in a reversible form of osteoporosis. This has recently been recognized as an iatrogenic phenomenon in the treatment of nodular thyroid glands with thyroxine, which may suppress TSH into the hyperthyroid range. Rheumatoid arthritis is a systemic catabolic illness with symmetrical arthritis. The resulting pain and stiffness in joints is associated with limited bone use and disuse osteoporosis. Renal tubular acidosis causes phosphaturia and hypophosphatemia, which results in the decreased mineralization of normal bone matrix known as osteomalacia. Polycystic ovarian syndrome is associated with obesity and usually mild androgenic abnormalities. Despite the lack of cyclic ovulatory menses, these women have steady-state estrogen secretion. These factors result in decreased risk of osteoporosis.

284–287. The answers are: 284-C, 285-A, 286-B, 287-E. *(Felig, ed 2. pp 1245–1280. Wilson, ed 12. pp 1814–1823.)* Lipoprotein disorders are now being described as specific apolipoprotein abnormalities that define the clinical entity. "Broad beta" disease, or type III hyperlipoproteinemia, is caused by critical changes in the amino acid sequence of apolipoprotein E. The result is accumulation of rem-nants of abnormal, very-low-density lipoproteins (VLDL). These remnants, display-ing a mobility on lipoprotein electrophoresis between prebeta- and betalipoproteins, present as a broad smear ("broad-beta band") between those two lipoprotein zones. On ultracentrifugation, however, the remnants sediment with VLDL. Plasma tri-glycerides and cholesterol are present in an approximate 1:1 ratio. The disorder is familial and associated with premature vascular disease. Planar xanthomas and tuberoeruptive xanthomas (confluent, eruptive lesions) of the elbows are virtually pathognomonic of broad-beta disease.

Familial defect in lipoprotein lipase can occur because of a genetic error in the enzyme or in apolipoprotein CII, which along with insulin activates lipoprotein lipase. The result is a failure to delipidate chylomicrons at the endothelial surface. The disorder usually appears in childhood, producing recurrent abdominal pain, pancreatitis, and signs of extreme elevations of triglycerides. The plasma will show a thick creamy layer on top and clear plasma below indicative of hyperchylomicronemia.

Disorders of the LDL receptor are inherited as a dominant trait. Afflicted heterozygous persons generally develop ischemic heart disease before the fifth decade of life. Clinical features include tendinous and tuberous xanthomas, arcus cornea, and occasionally xanthelasma. The disorder is a result of decreased receptor-mediated clearance of LDL. Increased production of VLDL can be induced by excessive caloric intake of alcohol, fat, or carbohydrates, or by conditions or agents that increase peripheral insulin resistance, such as diabetes mellitus, uremia, hydrochlorothiazides, glucocorticoids, or estrogens.

Increased levels of HDL are associated with reduced risk for atherosclerosis. HDL cholesterol levels are usually inversely related to triglyceride levels. The enhanced uptake of triglycerides from VLDL associated with exercise results in relative abundance of apolipoprotein C in the VLDL particle. This condition causes the apolipoprotein C to break off and transfer in the plasma to nascent HDL particles synthesized in the liver. The insertion of apolipoprotein C into nascent HDL results in a mature HDL, which has the capacity to pick up cholesterol in the periphery and transport the sterol to the liver for excretion or recycling.

288-291. The answers are: 288-D, 289-C, 290-A, 291-B. *(Felig, ed 2. pp 599-620, 1692-1698. Wilson, ed 12. pp 1718-1725, 1727-1729.)* Ectopic adrenocorticotropic hormone (ACTH) syndrome, as may be caused by oat cell carcinoma, is characterized by hypokalemic alkalosis, hyperpigmentation associated with elevated levels of ACTH, and myopathy. The characteristic clinical features of Cushing's syndrome are generally absent, probably because of the rapid development of the disorder. Urinary free cortisol, 17-hydroxycorticosteroids (OHCS), and 17-ketosteroids (KS), as well as plasma cortisol, are markedly elevated; dexamethasone fails to suppress 17-OHCS even when high doses are given.

Cushing's disease (pituitary-dependent bilateral adrenal hyperplasia) is characterized by the loss of diurnal variation in plasma cortisol, elevated urinary glucocorticoids and androgens, and the failure to suppress urinary free cortisol or 17-OHCS with the low-dose dexamethasone test. Plasma ACTH concentration is normal and mildly elevated and hypokalemic alkalosis is rarely present. Urinary 17-KS levels representing adrenal androgen production are increased in proportion to 17-OHCS since the glucocorticoid and the androgen producing zones of the adrenal gland are equally responsive to ACTH.

Patients who have adrenal carcinoma often display signs of excess adrenal androgen production that sometimes overshadow the signs of Cushing's syndrome.

Plasma cortisol and DHEA sulfate and urinary 17-KS may be dramatically increased; there is no 17-OHCS or 17-KS suppression even with the high-dose dexamethasone test. Characteristically, in adrenal carcinoma plasma ACTH is very low; in contrast, in Cushing's syndrome and ectopic ACTH syndrome, the ACTH levels are normal or increased.

Congenital adrenal hyperplasia results from a deficiency of one of several possible cortisol synthetic enzymes, the most common being 21-hydroxylase. Adrenal androgen production often is dramatically increased, while adrenal cortisol production may be normal or decreased. As a consequence of the excess androgen production, virilism occurs in the female and short stature is frequent in the male because of early closure of bony epiphyses. Urinary 17-KS levels are increased in congenital adrenal hyperplasia but are suppressed by dexamethasone. This feature distinguishes the disorder from adrenal tumors. Hyperpigmentation results from the compensatory increase in ACTH secretion.

Nelson's syndrome, which features marked hyperpigmentation and is caused by a pituitary macrotumor that appears after bilateral adrenalectomy for Cushing's disease, is disappearing as a clinical entity since transsphenoidal hypophysectomy is now the treatment of choice for the primary pituitary tumor.

292–296. The answers are: 292-B, 293-C, 294-B, 295-A, 296-A. (*Wilson, ed 12. pp 1811–1812.*) The components of MEN I are hyperparathyroidism, pancreatic islet cell tumors, and anterior pituitary tumors; tumors of the adrenal cortex and thyroid are less frequent features. The syndrome is inherited in an autosomal dominant fashion and presentations occur at any age. While asymptomatic hypercalcemia is common, 50 percent of patients have renal stones and 25 percent have osteitis fibrosa as manifestations of hyperparathyroidism. Most pancreatic islet cell tumors secrete gastrin or insulin and 10 percent of patients have complications of both. The diagnosis of gastrinomas rests on the demonstration of increased gastrin levels after secretin infusion, while insulinomas are characterized by fasting hypoglycemia coexistent with an elevated plasma insulin level. Islet cell tumors have the histologic appearance of carcinoid tumors. Pituitary tumors present either because of their size or because of their secretory capabilities; prolactinomas are the most common tumor type.

MEN II, in contrast, is characterized by medullary thyroid carcinoma, pheochromocytoma, and hyperparathyroidism; it is also transmitted in autosomal dominant fashion. Glandular involvement is typically multicentric as it is in MEN I. Medullary thyroid carcinoma is associated with early metastatic disease and multiple secretory products, the most common of which is calcitonin. Pheochromocytoma, the major cause of morbidity and mortality in patients with MEN II, typically develops at an older age and occurs as bilateral adrenal tumors in 60 to 70 percent of cases. These tumors manifest as hypertension and paroxysms of flushing, sweating, and headaches, or they may be asymptomatic. They are diagnosed by finding increased levels of catecholamines or catecholamine metabolites in a 24-h urine collection. Unlike patients with MEN I, most patients with MEN II and parathyroid hyperplasia are normocalcemic.

297–301.   The answers are: 297-A, 298-C, 299-C, 300-D, 301-D. *(Felig, ed 2. pp 432–435. Wilson, ed 12. p 1705.)* Hyperthyroidism results from the excessive secretion of thyroid hormones and is most commonly due to Graves' disease, thyroiditis, multinodular goiter, or thyroid adenoma. The choice of therapy, whether with antithyroid drugs, radiation, or surgery, is influenced by the patient's age and sex, status of the hyperthyroidism and cardiovascular system, and history of previous management of the disease.

The thionamide drugs used in the United States are propylthiouracil (PTU) and methimazole. Both drugs inhibit the incorporation of iodide into thyroglobulin by blocking iodine oxidation and organification and iodotyrosine coupling. They do not, however, block the release of previously formed and stored thyroid hormone. PTU has the advantage of inhibiting the extrathyroidal conversion of T_4 to T_3. Both drugs also have immunosuppressive activity: thyroid antibody production is inhibited, as are lymphocyte function and viability.

While the plasma half-life of PTU is 1 to 2 h and that of methimazole is 4 to 6 h, because the drugs are concentrated in the thyroid gland, serum levels do not reflect intrathyroidal concentrations.

Toxic reactions to these drugs occur in 5 to 10 percent of patients and most commonly consist of pruritus, urticaria, and other rashes; more serious side effects include fever, arthritis, vasculitis, hepatitis, anemia, and thrombocytopenia. In less than 0.5 percent of patients, a rapidly developing agranulocytosis occurs.

Gastroenterology

DIRECTIONS: Each question below contains five suggested responses. Select the **one best** response to each question.

302. All the following laboratory test abnormalities are poor prognostic factors in pancreatitis (Ranson criteria) EXCEPT

(A) significant decrease in hematocrit level
(B) hypocalcemia
(C) leukocytosis
(D) hyperglycemia
(E) steatorrhea

303. Primary biliary cirrhosis may produce all the following laboratory test results EXCEPT

(A) elevated serum immunoglobulin M (IgM)
(B) absent alpha₁ spike on serum protein electrophoresis (SPEP)
(C) elevated antimitochondrial antibody (AMA) titers
(D) hyperbilirubinemia
(E) elevated serum alkaline phosphatase level

304. Which one of the following clinical or laboratory findings is LEAST likely to occur in chronic pancreatitis?

(A) Steatorrhea
(B) Diabetes mellitus
(C) Pancreatic calcifications
(D) Bronzing of the skin
(E) Vitamin B_{12} malabsorption

305. In a patient who is seropositive for human immunodeficiency virus (HIV), all the following *intestinal* infections or tumors would be diagnostic of AIDS EXCEPT

(A) *Cryptosporidium* infection
(B) cytomegalovirus (CMV) infection
(C) tuberculosis
(D) *Mycobacterium avium-intracellulare* infection
(E) lymphoma

306. Which one of the following colonic polyps is most likely to be associated with colon cancer?

(A) Villous adenoma
(B) Tubular adenoma
(C) Hyperplastic polyp
(D) Lipoma
(E) Hamartoma

307. All the following ulcer characteristics or laboratory abnormalities would support the diagnosis of the Zollinger-Ellison syndrome EXCEPT

(A) elevated gastrin level
(B) multiple gastrointestinal ulcers
(C) gastrointestinal ulcers at unusual locations
(D) positive urease breath test
(E) positive (abnormal) secretin stimulation test

308. Crohn's disease is associated with an increased incidence of all the following EXCEPT

(A) kidney stones
(B) gallstones
(C) colon cancer
(D) porphyria cutanea tarda
(E) ankylosing spondylitis

309. All the following statements about achalasia are true EXCEPT

(A) the lower esophageal sphincter is hypertensive
(B) *Trypanosoma cruzi* may produce an achalasia-like illness
(C) the lower esophageal sphincter fails to relax with swallowing
(D) esophageal contraction waves are of low amplitude but are peristaltic
(E) it may be treated medically with nifedipine

DIRECTIONS: Each question below contains four suggested responses of which **one or more** is correct. Select

A	if	**1, 2, and 3**	are correct
B	if	**1 and 3**	are correct
C	if	**2 and 4**	are correct
D	if	**4**	is correct
E	if	**1, 2, 3, and 4**	are correct

310. Which of the following laboratory tests would typically be abnormal (positive) in a patient with celiac (nontropical) sprue?

(1) Small-bowel biopsy
(2) Fat content in 72-h stool collection
(3) D-Xylose test
(4) Secretin stimulation test

311. Vitamin B$_{12}$ (cyanocobalamin) deficiency may be produced by

(1) pernicious anemia
(2) Crohn's disease
(3) ileal resection
(4) chronic pancreatitis

312. Celiac disease (nontropical sprue) is associated with an increased incidence of

(1) gastrinoma
(2) lymphoma
(3) carcinoid
(4) dermatitis herpetiformis

313. Chronic pancreatitis frequently produces

(1) diabetes mellitus
(2) malabsorption of fat-soluble vitamins D and K
(3) steatorrhea
(4) Courvoisier's sign

314. Gastroenterologic cancers that have decreased in frequency over the past 50 years in the United States include

(1) colon cancer
(2) pancreatic cancer
(3) esophageal cancer
(4) gastric cancer

315. Correct statements about angiodysplasias (arteriovenous malformations) include that they

(1) can be diagnosed by air-contrast barium enema
(2) most frequently occur in the cecum
(3) most frequently occur in young adults
(4) are associated with aortic stenosis

316. The delta virus (hepatitis D) is known or believed to

(1) be an RNA-containing virus
(2) frequently be associated with a severe acute hepatitis
(3) require coinfection with hepatitis B
(4) be the most common cause of non-A, non-B hepatitis

317. Laboratory abnormalities associated with autoimmune hepatitis include

(1) antinuclear antibodies (ANA)
(2) hepatitis B surface antigen (HBsAg)
(3) anti-smooth muscle antibodies
(4) elevated serum immunoglobulin M (IgM) level

DIRECTIONS: Each group of questions below consists of lettered headings followed by a set of numbered items. For each numbered item select the **one** lettered heading with which it is **most** closely associated. Each lettered heading may be used **once, more than once, or not at all.**

Questions 318–321

For each histologic abnormality found on liver biopsy, select the liver disease with which it is associated.

(A) Schistosomiasis
(B) Primary biliary cirrhosis
(C) Alpha$_1$-antitrypsin deficiency
(D) Hemochromatosis
(E) Alcoholic hepatitis

318. Steatosis

319. Pipe-stem fibrosis

320. Paucity of bile ducts

321. PAS (periodic acid-Schiff)-positive granules

Questions 322–325

For each clinical finding occurring in patients with the acquired immunodeficiency syndrome (AIDS), choose the appropriate infectious agent.

(A) Herpes simplex virus
(B) *Cryptosporidium*
(C) Cytomegalovirus (CMV)
(D) *Candida*
(E) *Histoplasma capsulatum*

322. Giant esophageal ulcers

323. "Cheesy" exudate in the esophagus

324. Vesicles or small ulcers in the esophagus

325. Diarrhea

Questions 326–329

For each laboratory test or set of tests, choose the hepatobiliary disease in which it is most likely to be abnormal.

(A) Sclerosing cholangitis
(B) Primary biliary cirrhosis
(C) Autoimmune (lupoid) hepatitis
(D) Wilson's disease
(E) Hemochromatosis

326. Antinuclear antibodies (ANA)

327. Ceruloplasmin

328. Serum iron, total iron-binding capacity (TIBC), ferritin

329. Antimitochondrial antibodies (AMA)

Questions 330–333

For each of the listed forms of hepatic injury, select the medicinal agent most likely to cause this injury.

(A) Thorotrast (20% solution of thorium dioxide)
(B) Estrogens
(C) Methyldopa (Aldomet)
(D) 6-Mercaptopurine
(E) Chlorpromazine

330. Cholestasis

331. Hepatitis

332. Hepatic adenoma

333. Hepatic angiosarcoma

Questions 334–337

For each disease choose the laboratory test that would be most helpful in making the diagnosis.

(A) Bentiromide test
(B) Small-bowel series
(C) Small-bowel biopsy
(D) Endoscopic retrograde cholangiopancreatography (ERCP)
(E) Serum folate level

334. Sclerosing cholangitis

335. Blind loop syndrome

336. Celiac disease (nontropical sprue)

337. Chronic pancreatitis (pancreatic insufficiency)

Questions 338–341

For each of the following physical findings, select the liver disease with which it is most closely associated.

(A) Wilson's disease
(B) Alpha$_1$-antitrypsin disease
(C) Primary biliary cirrhosis
(D) Dubin-Johnson syndrome
(E) Hemochromatosis

338. Xanthomas

339. Sunflower cataracts

340. Bronzing of the skin

341. Kayser-Fleischer rings

Questions 342–345

Select the locations or ethnic groups that have a particularly high incidence of the diseases listed below.

(A) Japan
(B) Leningrad
(C) Mississippi River Valley
(D) Puma Indians
(E) Northeast Iran

342. Giardiasis

343. Histoplasmosis

344. Gastric cancer

345. Gallstones

Questions 346–349

For each clinical finding, select the appropriate gastrointestinal disease.

(A) Cholera
(B) Pancreatic cholera
(C) Salmonellosis
(D) Gastrinoma
(E) Shigellosis

346. Dysentery

347. Watery diarrhea and hypochlorhydria

348. Watery diarrhea without hypochlorhydria

349. Acidic diarrhea

Gastroenterology

Answers

302. The answer is E. *(Eastwood, pp 231–239.)* The Ranson criteria are used to gauge the severity of pancreatitis. The following abnormalities on admission, or within 2 days of admission, are associated with a worse prognosis: old age; leukocytosis; hyperglycemia; elevations of the serum LDH (lactate dehydrogenase), SGOT, or SGPT levels; hypoxemia; hypocalcemia; a declining hematocrit level; a significant base deficit; significant fluid sequestration; and hypoalbuminemia. Pancreatic insufficiency from chronic pancreatitis leads to steatorrhea.

303. The answer is B. *(Schiff, ed 6. pp 979–999.)* Primary biliary cirrhosis is a disease primarily affecting middle-aged women. Clinical findings include pruritus and elevated serum alkaline phosphatase and bilirubin levels. Patients with this disease characteristically develop antimitochondrial antibodies. Immunoelectrophoresis usually demonstrates an increase in the serum immunoglobulin M (IgM) levels. An absent alpha$_1$ spike on serum protein electrophoresis (SPEP) occurs in alpha$_1$-antitrypsin disease.

304. The answer is D. *(Eastwood, pp 240–247.)* Chronic pancreatitis results from chronic pancreatic damage. Because of inadequate production of pancreatic lipase, triglycerides are not enzymatically cleaved into free fatty acids and are malabsorbed. This results in steatorrhea, an elevated concentration of stool fat. The damaged pancreas may also produce insufficient insulin. Normally, R factors bind to ingested vitamin B$_{12}$ in the stomach; trypsin present in the duodenal lumen cleaves the R factors and permits intrinsic factor to bind to vitamin B$_{12}$ so that the vitamin can be absorbed in the terminal ileum. With pancreatic insufficiency, trypsin is not available, so that vitamin B$_{12}$ does not complex with intrinsic factor and is not absorbed. In contrast to other triglycerides, vitamin D is absorbed from the gastrointestinal tract intact without digestion by lipase. It is absorbed normally in patients with chronic pancreatitis. The scarred and fibrosed pancreas in chronic pancreatitis may develop calcifications.

305. The answer is A. *(Stein, ed 3. pp 1348–1350.)* Patients with HIV infection are at increased risk of developing severe infection with cytomegalovirus, tuberculosis, *Mycobacterium avium-intracellulare*, and *Cryptosporidium*. They are also at greatly increased risk of developing non-Hodgkin's lymphoma. Healthy patients may also develop an acute infection with *Cryptosporidium*. However, cryptosporidiosis for more than 1 month is diagnostic of AIDS. The other four diseases, when they involve the intestine, are diagnostic of AIDS.

306. The answer is A. *(Berk, ed 4. pp 2490-2516.)* Adenomas are benign tumors that may contain a focus of or develop into colon cancer. Villous adenomas are more likely than tubular adenomas to develop into colon cancer. Hamartomatous polyps are infrequently associated with colon cancer. Whether hyperplastic polyps have a malignant potential is controversial. Lipomas are not associated with colon cancer.

307. The answer is D. *(Sleisenger, ed 4. pp 909-925.)* The Zollinger-Ellison syndrome is characterized by a severe ulcer diathesis due to excessive gastrin production by a neurosecretory tumor that stimulates gastric hyperacidity. Multiple gastrointestinal ulcers frequently occur. Ulcers may occur at unusual locations, such as the esophagus and descending duodenum. The screening test for this disorder is a serum gastrin level obtained after an overnight fast. Pernicious anemia with atrophic gastritis or antral G cell hyperplasia can also produce an elevated gastrin level. A secretin test is used to differentiate between an elevated gastrin level due to a gastrinoma and one due to these other conditions. Elevation of the serum gastrin level by more than 200 pg/mL after intravenous administration of secretin is characteristic of a gastrinoma. The urease breath test is used to detect *Helicobacter* (previously *Campylobacter*) *pyloris* infection of the stomach. *Helicobacter pyloris* has been implicated as a cause of acute and chronic gastritis and may be associated with peptic ulcers.

308. The answer is D. *(Wilson, ed 12. pp 1268-1281.)* Crohn's disease is an idiopathic inflammatory bowel disease. Terminal ileitis produces a reduced bile salt pool. These abnormalities may produce steatorrhea and cholelithiasis. Normally dietary oxalate is bound by dietary calcium and not absorbed. When steatorrhea occurs, dietary calcium preferentially binds to free fatty acids and the unbound oxalic acid is absorbed. This may produce hyperoxaluria and renal oxalate stones. Crohn's disease is associated with an increased risk of developing ankylosing spondylitis and colon cancer. Porphyria cutanea tarda is associated with alcoholism and several medications.

309. The answer is D. *(Sleisenger, ed 4. pp 559-593.)* Achalasia is a disorder characterized by dysphagia due to abnormal esophageal motility. Esophageal manometry characteristically reveals the following abnormalities: First, the resting pressure of the lower esophageal sphincter is elevated. Second, the lower esophageal sphincter fails to relax with a swallow. Third, esophageal contractions with a swallow are *not* peristaltic. *Trypanosoma cruzi* infection may produce a secondary achalasia. Achalasia may be treated by administration of nifedipine, by esophageal pneumatic dilation, or by a Heller myotomy.

310.   The answer is A (1, 2, 3). *(Stein, ed 3. pp 295-296, 360-362.)* Celiac disease is caused by a reaction to gluten present in cereals. The pathologic examination of a small-bowel mucosal biopsy reveals flattened villi and intense mucosal inflammation. D-Xylose is absorbed by the enterocyte with no intraluminal digestion. D-Xylose is inadequately absorbed in celiac disease because of mucosal damage. In contrast, the D-xylose test is normal in pancreatic insufficiency. Celiac disease causes fat malabsorption and steatorrhea, which is proved by analysis of the total fat content in a 72-h collection of stool. Intravenous administration of secretin is used to analyze pancreatic function in suspected chronic pancreatitis and to determine whether a gastrinoma is present in a patient with a mildly elevated gastrin level.

311.   The answer is E (all). *(Eastwood, pp 161-162.)* Ingested vitamin B_{12} is first bound in the stomach to R factor proteins. In the duodenum, pancreatic enzymes cleave the R factors from vitamin B_{12}, permitting intrinsic factor to bind to the vitamin. Vitamin B_{12} bound to intrinsic factor is absorbed in the terminal ileum. The vitamin will not be absorbed in pernicious anemia because of an absence of intrinsic factor, after ileal resection or in Crohn's disease because of loss of the absorptive site, and in chronic pancreatitis because of a lack of pancreatic enzyme cleavage of the R factor.

312.   The answer is C (2, 4). *(Sleisenger, ed 4. pp 1134-1152.)* Celiac disease is an intestinal disease due to an abnormal intestinal reaction to ingested gluten in cereals. It is associated with an increased risk of lymphoma and of dermatitis herpetiformis.

313.   The answer is B (1, 3). *(Eastwood, pp 240-247.)* Chronic pancreatitis is due to pancreatic damage from recurrent attacks of acute pancreatitis. Pancreatic damage leads to deficient secretion of lipase and to steatorrhea. Insulin deficiency may result in diabetes mellitus. Vitamins D and K are absorbed intact from the intestines without digestion by lipase and are therefore absorbed normally in pancreatic insufficiency. Courvoisier's sign is a palpable, nontender gallbladder in a jaundiced patient. This finding suggests the presence of a malignancy, especially pancreatic cancer.

314.   The answer is D (4). *(Sleisenger, ed 4. pp 620, 750, 1519-1521, 1872-1873.)* In contrast to cancers of the colon, pancreas, and esophagus, gastric cancer has been decreasing in incidence in the United States. It has been hypothesized that this decrease may be related to less ingested carcinogens because of refrigeration of food.

315.   The answer is C (2, 4). *(Eastwood, pp 204-205.)* Angiodysplasias are arteriovenous communications or ectatic blood vessels. They frequently produce gastrointestinal bleeding in the elderly and are associated with aortic stenosis. Angiodysplasia may be diagnosed by angiography or colonoscopy but not by barium enema. The lesions are most commonly present in the cecum.

316. The answer is A (1, 2, 3). *(Zakim, ed 2. pp 916–920.)* The delta virus is a hepatotropic RNA-containing virus that requires coinfection with hepatitis B for replication. It can complicate acute or chronic hepatitis B infection. Delta virus infection tends to increase the severity of hepatitis B infection. Hepatitis C appears to be the most frequent cause of non-A, non-B hepatitis.

317. The answer is B (1, 3). *(Zakim, ed 2. pp 1032–1041.)* Autoimmune, or lupoid, hepatitis is an idiopathic autoimmune hepatic disease mostly affecting women. Patients develop high titers of antinuclear antibodies as in systemic lupus erythematosus (SLE). Also, patients may develop anti–smooth muscle antibodies, as occurs in other autoimmune diseases. An elevated serum IgM level occurs in primary biliary cirrhosis. HBsAg is present in hepatitis B infection.

318–321. The answers are: 318-E, 319-A, 320-B, 321-C. *(Sherlock, ed 8. pp 273–288, 491–493, 565–567. Wyngaarden, ed 18. pp 842–844.)* Alcoholic hepatitis typically presents with fever, pain and tenderness of the right upper quadrant, and hepatomegaly in an alcoholic patient. Typically the SGOT (serum glutamic oxaloacetic transaminase, AST) level is much higher than the SGPT (serum glutamic pyruvate transaminase, ALT) level. Although the diagnosis is usually made from these clinical findings, a liver biopsy would show prominent steatosis or fat.

The blood fluke *Schistosoma mansoni* invades the portal vessels, where it stimulates intense inflammation and fibrosis. The portal vessels become pipelike, hence, the name *pipe-stem fibrosis*. Schistosomiasis tends to produce portal hypertension with little derangement of liver function.

Primary biliary cirrhosis is a disease of unknown etiology primarily affecting females. The inflammatory destruction in this disease of small- and medium-sized bile ducts eventually produces a paucity of bile ducts in the late stage of the disease.

Alpha₁-antitrypsin disease is a genetic disease in which the normal trypsin inhibitor alpha₁-antitrypsin is not produced. Symptoms are produced by hepatic or pulmonic injury. The diagnosis is supported by an absence of the normal spike produced by alpha₁-globulins on serum protein electrophoresis. For a definitive diagnosis, the serum alpha₁-antitrypsin form is determined by electrophoresis or by monoclonal antibodies. Liver biopsy characteristically demonstrates intracellular granules that are stained by the periodic acid-Schiff reagent and resist digestion with diastase.

322–325. The answers are: 322-C, 323-D, 324-A, 325-B. *(Cappell, Am J Gastroenterol 86:1–15, 1991. Wilson, ed 12. pp 1402–1410.)* Cytomegalovirus typically produces a transient, self-limited illness in a healthy host. Patients with AIDS develop severe chronic infection that typically produces large or giant gastrointestinal ulcers.

Patients with AIDS frequently develop oral or esophageal candidiasis. Esophageal candidiasis typically produces odynophagia or dysphagia. The oropharyngeal or esophageal mucosa is covered by a cheesy white exudate. Pathologic examination of a biopsy will demonstrate the characteristic mycelial forms.

Herpes simplex type 1 produces in otherwise healthy patients vesicular lesions in the oropharynx, which then break down to form shallow ulcers prior to healing. Patients with AIDS may develop progressive, nonhealing vesicular or ulcerated lesions.

Cryptosporidium produces an acute, self-limited diarrheal illness in immunocompetent patients and a chronic, severe diarrheal illness in patients with AIDS. The diagnosis may be made by a small-bowel biopsy or by microscopic examination of fresh concentrated specimens of stool for ova and parasites with the use of a cold Kinyoun stain.

326–329. The answers are: 326-C, 327-D, 328-E, 329-B. *(Berk, ed 4. pp 3203–3235. Sherlock, ed 8. pp 273–288, 348–356.)* Autoimmune hepatitis was formerly called "lupoid hepatitis" because it shares some features with systemic lupus erythematosus (SLE), such as the presence of an elevated titer of serum antinuclear antibodies (ANA). This disease is treated by corticosteroids to reduce the immune-mediated hepatic injury.

Wilson's disease is a hereditary disease of copper metabolism manifested by pathologic deposition of copper in the liver, cornea, and brain. The serum ceruloplasmin level is almost always decreased with this disease. Another screening test is a slit-lamp ophthalmologic examination to detect the brown deposition on Descemet's membrane of the cornea, the Kayser-Fleischer rings.

Hemochromatosis is an autosomal recessive genetic disease of iron metabolism characterized by excessive iron absorption and abnormal iron storage within parenchymal organs, including the liver, pancreas, and heart. Hepatic deposition produces cirrhosis. With this disease, the serum ferritin level and the percentage of iron saturation (serum iron level divided by the total iron-binding capacity, expressed as a percentage) are abnormally elevated because of excessive bodily iron. This disease is usually diagnosed by a liver biopsy.

Primary biliary cirrhosis is an idiopathic hepatic disease primarily affecting small- or medium-sized bile ducts. It typically occurs in middle-aged females. Laboratory abnormalities include elevated serum alkaline phosphatase and bilirubin levels. Serum immunoelectrophoresis may demonstrate an elevated serum immunoglobulin M (IgM) level. Patients characteristically develop antimitochondrial antibodies.

330–333. The answers are: 330-E, 331-C, 332-B, 333-A. *(Zakim, ed 2. pp 754–791.)* Chlorpromazine, an antipsychotic medication, can produce cholestasis, manifested by an elevation of the serum alkaline phosphatase and bilirubin levels.

Patients may develop a flu-like syndrome and pruritus. Eosinophilia commonly occurs. Development of this side effect mandates discontinuation of this medication.

Methyldopa (Aldomet) is an antihypertensive medication that may produce an acute hepatitis with significant elevations of the serum glutamic oxaloacetic transaminase (SGOT, AST) and serum glutamic pyruvate transaminase (SGPT, ALT) levels. In most cases, cessation of administration leads to complete recovery, but occasionally chronic active hepatitis may occur.

Estrogens are frequently used in oral contraceptives. Adverse hepatic effects produced by estrogens include hepatic adenomas, focal nodular hyperplasia, and peliosis hepatis. Peliosis hepatis consists of abnormally dilated intraparenchymal vascular channels. Hepatic adenomas are benign tumors of hepatocytes. Estrogens have also been associated with the development of pancreatitis. Thorotrast, a 20% solution of thorium dioxide, was extensively used as a radiographic contrast material between 1930 and 1955. Unfortunately, it is never resorbed and continues to emit radioactive energy. This agent is no longer used because it has been associated with the development of angiosarcomas (hemangiosarcomas). Vinyl chloride workers are also at increased risk of developing this malignancy.

334–337.   The answers are: 334-D, 335-B, 336-C, 337-A. *(Berk, ed 4. pp 3177–3188. Eastwood, pp 240–247. Sleisenger, ed 4. pp 1134–1152, 1289–1297.)* Sclerosing cholangitis is a disorder of unknown etiology characterized by obstructed bile flow due to irregular beading and dilatation of the biliary tree. About 70 percent of cases are associated with ulcerative colitis. A sclerosing cholangitis-like illness has been reported in AIDS patients with biliary infection with cytomegalovirus and *Cryptosporidium*. The diagnosis is almost always made by radiographic observation of the bile ducts by endoscopic retrograde cholangiopancreatography (ERCP).

In the blind loop syndrome, small intestinal abnormalities such as diverticula, resection, adhesions, or fistulas create intestinal loops that drain poorly and permit bacterial overgrowth. The intestinal abnormalities may be detected by an upper gastrointestinal series with small-bowel follow-through or by a small-bowel series. Bacterial overgrowth may be demonstrated by a ^{14}C-xylose breath test or by a quantitative bacterial culture of a jejunal aspirate.

Celiac disease, or nontropical sprue, is caused by an immunologic reaction to gluten, which is a protein present in wheat. Microscopic examination of a mucosal small-bowel biopsy demonstrates blunting of the intestinal villi, lengthening of the mucosal crypts, and severe inflammation.

Pancreatic exocrine and endocrine insufficiency in chronic pancreatitis can result in diabetes mellitus and protein and fat malabsorption. Ingested bentiromide is normally cleaved by chymotrypsin in the intestine to liberate para-aminobenzoic acid (PABA), which is absorbed and excreted in the urine. Abnormally low recovery of PABA in the urine in a bentiromide test suggests decreased chymotrypsin secretion caused by pancreatic insufficiency.

338–341. The answers are: 338-C, 339-A, 340-E, 341-A. *(Sherlock, ed 8. pp 273–288, 460–469. Zakim, ed 2. pp 1273–1299.)* Primary biliary cirrhosis is a disease of unknown etiology primarily affecting middle-aged women. Impaired biliary excretion of cholesterol due to progressive bile duct damage leads to hypercholesterolemia and to cholesterol deposition as xanthelasma on the eyelids and xanthomas on the arms.

Excessive copper deposition leads to disease of the liver and basal ganglia in Wilson's disease. Ocular findings include the premature development of large cataracts, called sunflower cataracts, and deposition of a brown pigment in Descemet's membrane of the cornea, a phenomenon called Kayser-Fleischer rings.

Hemochromatosis is an inherited disease characterized by abnormally high iron absorption. Excessive iron is stored in the liver, pancreas, and heart. Subcutaneous iron deposition leads to bronzing of the skin.

342–345. The answers are: 342-B, 343-C, 344-A, 345-D. *(Sleisenger, ed 4. pp 745–772, 1153–1155, 1668–1714. Stein, ed 3. pp 1556–1562.)* Giardia lamblia, a protozoan, colonizes the proximal small bowel and produces diarrhea, abdominal discomfort, and bloating. The diagnosis may be missed by examination of the stool for ova and parasites; examination of a duodenal aspirate obtained at esophagogastroduodenoscopy (EGD) is the most sensitive test. Giardiasis is frequently transmitted by contaminated water. There is a high incidence of giardiasis in Leningrad.

Histoplasmosis is a common cause of a mild respiratory illness in endemic areas including the midwestern river valleys of the United States. Cave explorers or bird handlers are at high risk of developing the infection from infected birds. AIDS patients develop severe, extrapulmonic histoplasmosis.

Although the etiology of gastric cancer is unknown, it has been associated with dietary consumption of nitrates and nitrites. The Japanese have established screening programs for this disease because they are at very high risk of developing gastric cancer. Descendants of Japanese immigrants to America have a lower incidence of gastric cancer than native Japanese, which suggests that an environmental factor may be an important risk factor for developing this cancer.

Gallstones are classified as cholesterol stones; as pigment stones, which contain calcium bilirubinate; or as mixed stones, which contain both cholesterol and calcium bilirubinate. Risk factors for developing cholesterol gallstones are female sex, multiparity, obesity, age over 40, and hypercholesterolemia. American Indians are at a very high risk of developing cholesterol gallstones. Patients with hemolysis excrete excessive bilirubin, a breakdown product of heme, in their bile and therefore are at high risk of developing pigmented stones.

346–349. The answers are: 346-E, 347-B, 348-A, 349-D. *(Stein, ed 3. pp 337–338, 554–555, 1486–1488, 1495–1496.)* Shigellosis is a severe acute diarrheal disease produced by a gram-negative bacterium. It causes bacillary dysentery with intestinal ulceration and inflammation. The stool typically contains blood and mucus.

The clinical features of pancreatic cholera include severe watery diarrhea, hypokalemia, and achlorhydria due to secretion of vasoactive intestinal polypeptide (VIP) by a pancreatic tumor.

Vibrio cholerae, a noninvasive pathogen, produces a potent enterotoxin that stimulates adenylate cyclase production and intestinal secretion. The infection causes a severe watery, secretory diarrhea. The stool osmolarity is similar to that of plasma. Prompt replacement of fluid and electrolyte losses is an essential part of therapy.

A gastrinoma is a tumor that produces gastrin and causes the Zollinger-Ellison syndrome. Patients frequently develop peptic ulcers because gastrin stimulates gastric acid secretion. The large volume of gastric acid production may overwhelm the ability of intestinal secretions to neutralize the acid. An acidic diarrhea results from inactivation of pancreatic enzymes and damage to small intestinal mucosa from the hyperacidity.

Nephrology

DIRECTIONS: Each question below contains five suggested responses. Select the **one best** response to each question.

Questions 350–352

A patient's blood work shows the following: Na^+ 140 meq/L, K^+ 4.0 meq/L, BUN 28 mg/dL, glucose 180 mg/dL, and creatinine 2.0 mg/dL. A 24-h urine collection with a total volume of 1400 mL shows a urine creatinine of 100 mg/dL and urine Na^+ of 70 meq/L.

350. Which of the following is a reasonable estimate of this patient's glomerular filtration rate? (Assume 1 day = 1400 min.)

(A) 50 mL/min
(B) 70 mL/min
(C) 100 mL/min
(D) 200 mL/min
(E) 700 mL/min

351. The fractional excretion of Na^+ (FE_{Na}) is

(A) 1.0 percent
(B) 2.5 percent
(C) 5.0 percent
(D) 10 percent
(E) 50 percent

352. Which of the following is the best estimate of this patient's serum osmolality? (Assume Na^+, its accompanying anion, BUN [molecular weight 28], and glucose [molecular weight 180] are the major contributors.)

(A) 140 mOsm/kg
(B) 200 mOsm/kg
(C) 300 mOsm/kg
(D) 488 mOsm/kg
(E) 1000 mOsm/kg

353. You are asked to evaluate a patient in the emergency room. He was brought by the rescue squad in a comatose state. Serum electrolytes drawn on admission show the following: Na^+ 133, K^+ 8.0, Cl^- 98, HCO_3^- 13. An electrocardiogram shows a rhythm with absence of P waves, a widened QRS complex, and peaked T waves. Which would be the most appropriate initial step?

(A) Repeat electrolyte measurements and observe

(B) Attempt cardioversion

(C) Administer intravenous calcium gluconate

(D) Administer hydrochlorothiazide, 25 mg orally

(E) Administer intravenous potassium chloride, 20 meq over 1 h

DIRECTIONS: Each question below contains four suggested responses of which **one or more** is correct. Select

A	if	**1, 2, and 3**	are correct
B	if	**1 and 3**	are correct
C	if	**2 and 4**	are correct
D	if	**4**	is correct
E	if	**1, 2, 3, and 4**	are correct

354. Treatment of hypertension in pregnancy can be safely accomplished using

(1) methyldopa (Aldomet)
(2) captopril
(3) hydralazine
(4) nitroprusside

355. Glomerulonephritides associated with depressed levels of serum complement include

(1) postinfectious glomerulonephritis (e.g., poststreptococcal glomerulonephritis)
(2) membranoproliferative glomerulonephritis
(3) lupus nephritis
(4) IgA nephropathy

356. Multiple myeloma may be associated with

(1) hypercalcemia
(2) the Fanconi syndrome
(3) distal renal tubular acidosis
(4) low anion gap

357. True statements concerning vitamin D include

(1) 25 (OH) vitamin D is the most active form
(2) 1,25 $(OH)_2$ vitamin D stimulates the resorption of calcium from bone
(3) 1,25 $(OH)_2$ vitamin D decreases the absorption of phosphorus from the GI tract
(4) 1,25 $(OH)_2$ vitamin D increases the absorption of calcium from the GI tract

358. True statements regarding polyarteritis nodosa (PAN) include which of the following?

(1) Renal arteriography can be helpful in the diagnosis of "classic" (macroscopic) PAN
(2) Hypertension is rare in classic PAN
(3) PAN may be associated with high titers of antineutrophilic cytoplasmic antibody (ANCA)
(4) Steroid therapy is felt to be ineffective in PAN

DIRECTIONS: Each group of questions below consists of lettered headings followed by a set of numbered items. For each numbered item select the **one** lettered heading with which it is **most** closely associated. Each lettered heading may be used **once, more than once, or not at all**.

Questions 359–362

Match each patient with the most likely renal calculi.

(A) Calcium oxalate stones
(B) Struvite (triple-phosphate) stones
(C) Cystine stones
(D) Uric acid stones

359. Patient with a myeloproliferative disorder

360. Patient with Crohn's disease

361. Patient with recurrent urinary tract infections by *Proteus* species

362. A 20-year-old man with recurrent stones; urinalysis shows many hexagonal crystals

Questions 363–366

In the following patients with the nephrotic syndrome, choose the likely finding on renal biopsy.

(A) Focal and segmental areas of mesangial sclerosis
(B) Diffuse mesangial deposition of acidophilic material with green birefringence on Congo red staining
(C) Normal glomeruli on light microscopy (LM) with fusion of foot processes noted on electron microscopy (EM)
(D) Diffuse thickening of the glomerular basement membrane on LM with subepithelial dense deposits on EM

363. A 4-year-old child with proteinuria

364. A patient treated with penicillamine for 10 months

365. A 28-year-old HIV-positive patient

366. A patient with familial Mediterranean fever

Questions 367–370

Match the set of electrolytes and blood gases most compatible with the clinical setting below.

| | Serum Electrolytes (meq/L) | | | | Arterial Blood Gas | | Urinary |
	Na	K	Cl	HCO$_3$	pH	P$_{CO_2}$ (mmHg)	Chloride (meq/L)
(A)	136	3.2	90	37	7.51	48	5
(B)	138	3.1	113	16	7.32	32	–
(C)	135	5.5	100	8	7.20	20	–
(D)	143	2.9	97	36	7.50	47	50

367. Patient with diarrhea

368. Patient with diabetic ketoacidosis

369. Patient with vomiting

370. Patient with mineralocorticoid excess from an adrenal tumor

---

Questions 371–373

Match the diuretic with the physiologic properties noted below.

(A) Increases reabsorption of calcium
(B) Inhibits the Na$^+$/K$^+$/2Cl$^-$ carrier along the thick ascending loop of Henle
(C) May induce a metabolic acidosis
(D) Commonly causes hyperkalemia
(E) None of the above

371. Furosemide

372. Acetazolamide

373. Hydrochlorothiazide

DIRECTIONS: The group of questions below consists of four lettered headings followed by a set of numbered items. For each numbered item select

A   if the item is associated with   (A) **only**
B   if the item is associated with   (B) **only**
C   if the item is associated with   **both** (A) and (B)
D   if the item is associated with   **neither** (A) nor (B)

Each lettered heading may be used **once, more than once, or not at all.**

Questions 374–377

(A) Prerenal azotemia
(B) Acute tubular necrosis (ATN)
(C) Both
(D) Neither

374.   Urine osmolality of 600 mOsm/kg

375.   Rising BUN and creatinine

376.   Urine sodium of 80 meq/L

377.   Urinalysis showing many tubular epithelial cells, granular casts, and tubular epithelial cell casts

Nephrology
Answers

350-352.   The answers are: 350-A, 351-A, 352-C. *(Rose, Clinical Physiology, ed 3. pp 61-68, 592-593. Rose, Pathophysiology, ed 2. p 68.)* Glomerular filtration rate (GFR) can best be determined by measuring the clearance of a compound (at steady state) that is freely filtered at the level of the glomerulus, is not protein-bound, and is neither secreted nor reabsorbed by the tubules. Therefore, for this compound (C):

$$\text{Amount of C filtered} = \text{amount excreted}$$
$$P_c \times \text{GFR} = U_c \times V$$
$$\text{GFR} = \frac{U_c \times V}{P_c} \text{ (clearance of C)}$$

Where P_c = plasma concentration of C, U_c = urine concentration of C, V = urine volume. Inulin meets all the above criteria. Determination of inulin clearance, however, can be cumbersome. Therefore, creatinine (Cr) clearance is usually used. The daily production of Cr is relatively constant. It is filtered freely at the glomerulus and not reabsorbed by the tubule (though 10 to 20 percent of the urinary creatinine does come from proximal tubular secretion). Therefore, for this patient:

$$\text{GFR} = \frac{U_{Cr} \times V}{P_{Cr}} = \frac{100 \text{ mg/dL} \times 14 \text{ dL (1400 mL)}}{2 \text{ mg/dL}} = 700 \text{ dL/day}$$

The GFR is then determined by converting to milliliters per minute:
$$700 \text{ dL/day} = 70{,}000 \text{ mL/1400 min} = 50 \text{ mL/min}$$

Measurement of the fractional excretion of sodium (FE_{Na}) can be helpful in distinguishing between prerenal azotemia and acute tubular necrosis (particularly in the oliguric patient). A low FE_{Na} reflects the sodium retention typical of prerenal states. FE_{Na} is the percentage of sodium (Na) filtered at the glomerulus and ultimately excreted in the urine.

$$FE_{Na} = \frac{Na \text{ excreted}}{Na \text{ filtered}} = \frac{U_{Na} \times V}{P_{Na} \times GFR} = \frac{U_{Na} \times V}{P_{Na} \times \dfrac{U_{Cr} \times V}{P_{Cr}}}$$

$$= \frac{U_{Na}/P_{Na}}{U_{Cr}/P_{Cr}} \quad or \quad \frac{U_{Na} \times P_{Cr}}{P_{Na} \times U_{Cr}}$$

$$= \frac{70 \times 2}{140 \times 100} \times 100 = 1.0 \text{ percent}$$

Plasma osmolality is a reflection of milliosmoles (mOsm) of solute per kilogram (kg) of water. The major contributors to osmolality include sodium, its accompanying anions (primarily Cl^- and HCO_3^-), BUN, and glucose. Since BUN and glucose are generally measured in milligrams per deciliter (mg/dL), one has to convert to milliequivalents per kilogram (meq/kg). This can be done by multiplying by 10 and dividing by the molecular weight:

$$Plasma \text{ osmolality} = 2 \times Na + \frac{glucose \times 10}{180} + \frac{BUN \times 10}{28}$$

$$= 2 \times Na + \frac{glucose}{18} + \frac{BUN}{2.8}$$

$$= 2 \times 140 + \frac{180}{18} + \frac{28}{2.8}$$

$$= 300 \text{ mOsm/kg}$$

353. The answer is C. *(Rose, Clinical Physiology, ed 3. pp 757–790.)* This patient presents with severe hyperkalemia. Although potassium elevations can occasionally be spurious (e.g., in hemolysis) the changes on this patient's ECG reflect severe cardiotoxic effects from the hyperkalemia. The ECG shows a typical progression in hyperkalemia with peaked T waves followed by widening of the QRS, loss of P waves, and eventually a sine wave pattern. Therapy of severe hyperkalemia includes intravenous calcium gluconate (to normalize membrane excitability), glucose and insulin, and sodium bicarbonate (to drive potassium intracellularly), and potassium exchange resins (to remove potassium). Dialysis may occasionally be necessary, particularly in patients with concomitant renal failure.

354.   The answer is B (1, 3). *(Rose, Pathophysiology, ed 2. p 347.)* Hypertension in pregnancy, whether it be preeclampsia or chronic hypertension exacerbated by pregnancy, can be a difficult therapeutic problem. In general, the time-tested drugs include methyldopa and hydralazine. The beta-adrenergic blockers are also being commonly used and except for occasional side effects, such as fetal bradycardia and hypoglycemia, they appear to be fairly safe. Nitroprusside and the angiotensin converting enzyme inhibitors (e.g., captopril) have been associated with fetal demise (the former thought to be secondary to cyanide poisoning) and, therefore, should not be used. Diuretics probably should be avoided, particularly in preeclampsia, as circulating volume is generally reduced in this condition. Ganglionic blockers and clonidine are not recommended.

355.   The answer is A (1, 2, 3). *(Rose, Pathophysiology, ed 2. p 166.)* When hypocomplementemia occurs in association with glomerulonephritis, the differential diagnostic list may be narrowed considerably. Specific entities include lupus nephritis, mixed cryoglobulinemia, membranoproliferative glomerulonephritis (MPGN), and postinfectious glomerulonephritis (including poststreptococcal glomerulonephritis, bacterial endocarditis, and the nephritis associated with infected ventriculoatrial shunts). Low levels of complements often result from increased degradation, which in some cases of MPGN may be secondary to the stabilization of C3 convertase by a circulating autoantibody (C3 nephritic factor). IgA nephropathy does not typically present with hypocomplementemia.

356.   The answer is E (all). *(Massry, ed 2. pp 738–745. Smolens, Am Kidney Fund Nephrol Lett, vol 4, no 4, 1987.)* Myeloma can be associated with a variety of electrolyte and renal tubular abnormalities. Hypercalcemia is a fairly common finding and is felt to occur secondary to the release of factors such as osteoclastic activating factors (OAF), which stimulate bone resorption. Occasionally these patients may also present with pseudohypercalcemia caused by high levels of calcium-binding paraproteins. In this case, patients are typically asymptomatic because the levels of ionized calcium are normal. Among the tubular defects reported with myeloma, distal renal tubular acidosis, nephrogenic diabetes insipidus, and the Fanconi syndrome are commonly mentioned. These defects are felt to be secondary to direct toxic effects of the light chains (particularly kappa) on the proximal or distal tubules or both. The low anion gap occasionally seen in myeloma (mainly IgG myeloma) is secondary to large amounts of circulating, positively charged paraproteins, which serve as unmeasured cations. (The formula for the anion gap can be derived as follows: since electrical neutrality must be maintained, Na^+ + unmeasured cations = Cl^- + HCO_3^- + unmeasured anions; hence, anion gap = Na^+ - (Cl^- + HCO_3^-) = unmeasured anions - unmeasured cations.) Therefore an increase in unmeasured cations lowers the anion gap. Patients whose paraprotein is negatively charged (such as those with IgA myeloma) should not have a low anion gap unless levels of albumin are very low (because albumin serves as an unmeasured anion).

357. The answer is C (2, 4). *(Holic, Kidney Int 32:912-929, 1987. Massry, ed 2. pp 193-201.)* Vitamin D_3 is synthesized in the skin through the effect of sunlight on 7-dehydrocholesterol. It subsequently undergoes hydroxylation in the liver and kidney to form, respectively, 25 (OH) vitamin D_3 and 1,25 (OH)$_2$ vitamin D_3. The latter dihydroxy form is the activated form of the vitamin. 1,25 (OH)$_2$ vitamin D_3 (DHVD) has a variety of biologic functions including maintaining calcium homeostasis. It stimulates both calcium and phoshorus absorption in the intestine and the resorption of calcium from bone. The latter function is felt to be mediated partially by DHVD's stimulating monocytes to become osteoclasts. Recently, various other interesting properties of DHVD have been elucidated, including immunomodulatory effects on B and T lymphocytes, and possible regulatory effects on insulin release.

358. The answer is B (1, 3). *(Balow, Kidney Int 27:954-964, 1985. Massry, ed 2. pp 707-714.)* Polyarteritis nodosa (PAN) is a form of systemic vasculitis in which renal involvement is frequent. In the "classic," or macroscopic, form of the disease, medium to small arteries are affected predominantly. Renal damage is felt to be secondary to parenchymal ischemia or infarction, which often leads to a renin-mediated hypertension. Inflammation of the blood vessel leads to aneurysm formation secondary to destruction of the lamina elastica. Demonstration of such aneurysmal dilatation on renal, mesenteric, or hepatic arteriography can be very helpful in confirming the diagnosis. Microsopic PAN involves predominantly the small vessels (capillaries, venules, and arterioles). Hypertension is relatively uncommon; however, glomerular involvement (i.e., glomerulonephritis) is frequent. Laboratory findings may be nonspecific. An elevated sedimentation rate is often noted. Recently, a new serologic marker has been discovered that is elevated in various forms of the vasculitides (particularly Wegener's granulomatosis and microscopic PAN). Antibodies to neutrophilic cytoplasmic antigens (ANCA) appear to be a fairly specific and sensitive test in the diagnosis of renal vasculitis. Hepatitis B antigen, rheumatoid factor, and cryoglobulins also have been reported in patients with PAN. The use of glucocorticoid therapy (with and without cytotoxics) has improved long-term prognosis.

359-362.   The answers are: 359-D, 360-A, 361-B, 362-C. *(Massry, ed 2. pp 920-941.)* Nephrolithiasis is becoming an increasingly prevalent problem in Western society. Patients with renal stones often present with signs of partial or complete obstruction, flank or abdominal pain, and hematuria. Calcium oxalate (alone or in combination with apatite) stones are by far the most common, accounting for approximately three-quarters of all stones. They are typically radiodense and therefore can often be detected on plain abdominal films. Hypercalciuria (with or without hypercalcemia), hyperoxaluria, hyperuricosuria, decreased urinary citrate, and decreased urine volumes can all predispose to calcium oxalate precipitation. Hyperoxaluria can either be primary (i.e., an inherited enzyme defect) or acquired. The most common cause of the latter is the increased intestinal absorption of oxalate in patients with small intestinal bypass or inflammatory bowel disease (such as Crohn's disease).

Struvite (triple-phosphate) stones are most commonly seen in patients with recurrent infections with uricase-producing bacteria (such as *Proteus*). Uricase-driven conversion of urea to ammonia and CO_2 (and eventually NH_4^+ and HCO_3^-) supports a persistently alkaline urine (pH greater than 7.5), which favors the formation of struvite ($MgNH_4PO_4 \cdot 6H_2O$) crystals. These stones are also radiopaque and occasionally can become quite large within the renal pelvis and calyces (so called staghorn calculi).

Uric acid stones account for 5 to 10 percent of all stones. In contrast to calcium oxalate and struvite, these stones are usually radiolucent. Hyperuricemia and attendant hyperuricosuria (such as is seen in myeloproliferative disorders, or with defects of purine synthesis) can predispose to uric acid stones. Acid urine and low urine volumes also favor stone formation. Raising urine (pH) to above 6.0 to 6.5 can be very effective in solubilizing uric acid.

Cystine stones are relatively rare and occur in patients with an inherited disorder of amino acid handling resulting in excessive urinary excretion of cystine, ornithine, lysine, and arginine. The urinalysis often shows the distinctive hexagon-shaped cystine crystals.

363-366.   The answers are: 363-C, 364-D, 365-A, 366-B. *(Rose, Pathophysiology, ed 2. pp 179-296.)* In each of the listed cases, the patient is presenting with the nephrotic syndrome (NS). NS can be defined as urinary protein excretion of greater than or equal to 3.0 to 3.5 g/day (in the adult) usually associated with edema, low levels of albumin, and hyperlipidemia. Proteinuria of this degree almost always indicates glomerular pathology.

When evaluating a patient with glomerulopathy, a routine urinalysis (UA) can be very helpful in selecting a differential diagnostic set. Conditions such as minimal change disease, focal segmental glomerular sclerosis, diabetes, membranous nephropathy, amyloidosis, and preeclampsia are usually associated with a nephrotic sediment with heavy proteinuria and little in the way of cellular elements or casts. On the other hand, a nephritic sediment (such as seen with proliferative nephritis) typically contains many red blood cells, often with red blood cell or granular casts with variable amounts of proteinuria.

The most common cause of NS in children is minimal change disease, which represents up to 90 percent of cases. The UA routinely shows proteinuria, with microscopic hematuria present in a minority of cases. On biopsy the glomeruli usually appear normal on light microscopy. The diagnosis is confirmed by electron microscopy, which shows fusion of the epithelial foot processes. Response to steroids is quite good, with the great majority of the children having a complete remission by 5 to 8 weeks. Relapses, however, are very common and can be treated with recurrent steroid therapy or, for those with very frequent relapses, cytotoxic agents.

In adults, membranous nephropathy (MN) is the most frequent cause of idiopathic nephrotic syndrome. The majority of patients with MN have no discernible cause. However, in approximately one-third of the patients, a causative disorder such as chronic hepatitis B infection, malignancy, or certain drugs can be identified. Drugs associated with MN include gold and penicillamine. Pathology may vary according to the stage of the disease, but typically manifests diffuse thickening of the glomerular basement membrane with subepithelial dense deposits on EM. Immunofluorescence (IF) usually shows diffuse granular deposits of IgG and C3.

Focal segmental glomerulosclerosis (FSGS) accounts for approximately 10 to 15 percent of the cases of nephrotic syndrome. Again, the majority of the cases of FSGS are idiopathic, though occasionally a secondary cause can be elicited, such as chronic reflux nephropathy, chronic renal transplant rejection, heroin use, and most recently HIV (AIDS) nephropathy. FSGS is the most common cause of nephrotic syndrome in patients with AIDS and appears to take a particularly aggressive course. Renal biopsy usually shows focal (involvement of some glomeruli) and segmental (involvement of some glomerular capillary loops) areas of sclerosis often associated with deposits of IgM and C3. Epithelial foot process fusion is noted on EM.

Amyloidosis, either primary or secondary, very frequently involves the kidneys. In primary (AL) amyloidosis there is increased production of, and tissue deposition of, fragments of monoclonal light chains (presumably from abnormal plasma cells). Chronic inflammation (from conditions such as rheumatoid arthritis and familial Mediterranean fever) can lead to secondary (AA) amyloidosis partially by the stimulation of secretion of serum amyloid A protein by the liver. Pathologically, one notes diffuse deposition of amorphous acidophilic material within the mesangium, the capillaries, and occasionally the vessels and tubules. These deposits show a characteristic green birefringence with Congo red staining. The presence of typical fibrils of amyloid proteins on EM confirms the diagnosis.

367-370.   The answers are: 367-B, 368-C, 369-A, 370-D. *(Rose, Clinical Physiology, ed 3. pp 464-477, 478-555.)* Changes in concentration of serum hydrogen ion are reflected by a reciprocal change in extracellular pH ($-\log[H^+]$, normal values 7.37 to 7.43). *Primary* metabolic acidosis and alkalosis result from a decrease or increase in serum bicarbonate, respectively. The respiratory compensation in these cases acts to return pH toward normal (by decreasing P_{CO_2} in the case of a metabolic acidosis or increasing P_{CO_2} in the case of metabolic alkalosis).

Metabolic alkalosis is associated with an elevated serum HCO_3^- and pH, and a compensatory rise in P_{CO_2}. This can result from a gain of HCO_3^- or from loss of hydrogen ions. To maintain the alkalosis, however, the renal tubules must reclaim the generated bicarbonate (the stimulus for which is often provided by concomitant factors such as volume depletion, chloride depletion, potassium depletion, and mineralocorticoid excess). Metabolic alkalosis associated with volume depletion (from conditions such as vomiting and distant diuretic use) is usually reflected by a urinary chloride of less than 15 meq/L. The metabolic alkalosis noted in primary mineralocorticoid excess states will usually be associated with a urinary chloride greater than 20 meq/L.

Metabolic acidosis is associated with a fall in HCO_3^- concentration, low blood pH, and compensatory decline in P_{CO_2}. Metabolic acidosis results from a gain of hydrogen ions, loss of HCO_3^- ions or the inability of the kidney to excrete the 1 to 1.5 meq/kg per day of hydrogen ions normally generated by the body. Conditions such as lactic acidosis or diabetic ketoacidosis, in which the bicarbonate is replaced by an unmeasured anion (e.g., lactate, beta-hydroxybutyrate), will be associated with a rise in the anion gap (normal 9 to 14). Remember that the anion gap = Na^+ - (Cl^- + HCO_3^-). Therefore, in conditions such as diarrhea or renal tubular acidoses, in which Cl rises as HCO_3^- falls, the anion gap will not be elevated. Common causes of high-anion-gap and normal-anion-gap acidoses are listed below:

High-anion-gap acidosis	Normal-anion-gap acidosis
—Lactic acidosis	—Diarrhea
—Ketoacidosis (diabetic, alcoholic)	—Renal tubular acidosis
—Ingestions	Type I (distal)
Ethylene glycol	Type II (proximal)
Methanol	Type IV (hyporenin,
Salicylates	hypoaldosterone states)
Paraldehyde	—Ammonium chloride
—Renal failure (usually late)	—Ureterosigmoidostomy
	—Carbonic anhydrase inhibitors
	—Chronic renal disease

371–373. The answers are: 371-B, 372-C, 373-A. *(Rose, Clinical Physiology, ed 3. pp 389–415.)* Diuretics enhance salt excretion by inhibiting NaCl reabsorption at various tubular sites. Acetazolamide, by inhibiting carbonic anhydrase, decreases Na^+, Cl^-, and HCO_3^- reclamation along the proximal tubule. The ensuing loss of alkali (as $NaHCO_3$) can evoke a metabolic acidosis. Acetazolamide, however, is a relatively weak diuretic, partially because of the ability of more distal sites to increase solute reabsorption.

The loop diuretics (furosemide, bumetanide, and ethacrynic acid) are the most potent diuretics. They inhibit the $Na^+/K^+/2Cl^-$ transporter along the loop of Henle. These agents also inhibit calcium reabsorption at this site and thereby increase calcium excretion.

The thiazide diuretics inhibit Na^+ and Cl^- reabsorption along the distal tubule (and connecting segment) and induce a modest natriuresis. Contrary to the loop diuretics, these agents increase calcium reabsorption, presumably both by a direct distal effect and at the proximal tubule (owing to volume depletion).

374–377. The answers are: 374-A, 375-C, 376-B, 377-B. *(Rose, Pathophysiology, ed 2. pp 63–117.)* When evaluating a patient with worsening renal function (i.e., rising BUN/creatinine), it is important to localize the pathology to a prerenal, intrinsic renal, or postrenal (obstructive) process. Obstruction must be ruled out in any patient presenting with azotemia. This can usually be done by bladder catheterization and renal ultrasound. The distinction between prerenal azotemia and acute tubular necrosis (a common cause of intrinsic renal failure in hospitalized patients) can be more difficult, and one has to rely on laboratory tests and urinary indices (particularly helpful in the oliguric patient) to help with the diagnosis.

Prerenal azotemia reflects a state of decreased renal perfusion. This can occur from frank volume depletion (such as with diarrhea) or with decreased effective circulating volume (such as with congestive heart failure). Under these conditions, the renal tubules react appropriately to the exogenous insult by reabsorbing water and avidly retaining sodium, thus excreting a concentrated urine (osmolality usually > 500 mOsm/kg) essentially devoid of sodium (usually < 20 meq/L). The urinalysis in this situation is typically bland without much in the way of cellular elements.

With ischemic or nephrotoxic injury to the kidneys (the main causes of ATN), the ability of the damaged tubules to concentrate urine and reabsorb sodium is significantly reduced. This will be reflected by a high urinary sodium (usually > 40 meq/L) and a urine osmolality approaching that of plasma. The urinalysis in ATN often shows many granular casts, tubular epithelial cells, and tubular epithelial cell casts.

Calculation of the fractional excretion of sodium (FE_{Na}) is also helpful. Prerenal states are usually associated with a FE_{Na} of less than 1 percent and ATN with FE_{Na} greater than 2 percent.

These indices are general guidelines and should be interpreted in concert with a careful history, physical examination, and other laboratory values.

Oncology and Hematology

DIRECTIONS: Each question below contains four or five suggested responses. Select the **one best** response to each question.

378. Heparin is a naturally occurring mucopolysaccharide that binds to antithrombin III and transforms this molecule into a potent inhibitor of thrombin and other serine proteases. Complications of heparin anticoagulation include all the following EXCEPT

(A) vertebral body collapse
(B) hemorrhage
(C) thrombosis
(D) skin necrosis
(E) thrombocytopenia

379. Marrow ablative-dose chemotherapy or chemoradiotherapy followed by bone marrow transplantation may be curative in leukemia, lymphoma, and possibly other malignancies. Which of the following diseases may be cured only by ablative therapy and bone marrow transplantation?

(A) Acute lymphoblastic leukemia (ALL)
(B) Acute myelogenous leukemia (AML)
(C) Chronic myelogenous leukemia (CML)
(D) Large cell lymphoma (LCL)

380. Sickle cell disease arises from the homozygous inheritance of a variant gene for beta globin resulting in a single amino acid substitution (valine replaces glutamic acid at the sixth position). Sickle beta globin undergoes concentration-dependent intracellular polymerization and sickling with loss of red cell deformability leading to hemolysis and vascular occlusive events. All the following statements regarding this disease are true EXCEPT

(A) sudden overwhelming infection may complicate the disease
(B) differentiation of crisis pain from other processes is possible by clinical laboratory studies
(C) hydration and analgesia represent basic management of painful crisis
(D) heterozygotes for Hgb S have a decreased risk from malaria, which may account for the prevalence of Hgb S
(E) exchange or hypertransfusion is indicated in children who have had a stroke

381. Oncogenes are important in at least some and perhaps many types of cancer. All the following statements regarding oncogenes are true EXCEPT

(A) oncogenes can be identified in the DNA of less than 60 percent of normal persons
(B) RNA retroviruses may induce oncogenesis by interfering with normal control mechanisms or by inserting transforming viral oncogenes
(C) infection with the human T-cell lymphotropic virus, type I (HTLV-I retrovirus), is associated with T-cell leukemia endemic in Japan, the Caribbean, and the southeastern U.S.
(D) chromosomal translocation may result in cancer by altering regulation and expression of cellular proto-oncogenes

382. Vitamin B_{12} deficiency and therapy are characterized by all the following statements EXCEPT

(A) neurologic symptoms may precede anemia
(B) only the first stage of the Schilling test is abnormal in patients with bacterial overgrowth
(C) hypokalemia may develop during initial replacement therapy
(D) erythroid hyperplasia is characteristic in megaloblastosis
(E) reticulocytosis occurs on the third to fifth day after inital vitamin B_{12} replacement

383. Severe aplastic anemia is associated with a granulocyte level < 500 cells per microliter, a platelet count of $< 20,000$, and a reticulocyte count less than 1 percent in association with profound marrow hypocellularity. All the following statements are true EXCEPT

(A) hepatitis is associated with aplastic anemia
(B) before effective treatment was available for severe aplastic anemia, mortality at 12 months following diagnosis was greater than 50 percent
(C) allogeneic bone marrow transplant (BMT) is the treatment of choice in younger patients
(D) aggressive immunosuppressive therapy may achieve remission in lupus, but not in chloramphenicol-related aplasia
(E) blood product transfusion may impair engraftment

384. Myelophthisic anemias are characterized by a peripheral blood smear containing all the following EXCEPT

(A) giant platelets
(B) spur cells (acanthocytes)
(C) nucleated red cells
(D) immature granulocytes
(E) teardrop cells (dacryocytes)

385. A 57-year-old man is found on physical examination to be plethoric with splenomegaly in the absence of cardiac or pulmonary disease. Laboratory examination reveals a hematocrit of 62 percent, a white cell count of 24,000/mm³, and thrombocytosis. Red blood cell mass is elevated as determined by isotope dilution. True statements concerning this patient's condition include each of the following EXCEPT

(A) 2 percent of patients without prior therapy experience transformation to acute leukemia
(B) there is an increased incidence of peptic ulcer disease
(C) a cerebrovascular event is a common complication
(D) urine levels of erythropoietin are substantially elevated
(E) pruritus, particularly after bathing, is a frequent complaint

386. All the following drugs are contraindicated in patients with glucose-6-phosphate dehydrogenase deficiency EXCEPT

(A) sulfapyridine
(B) nitrofurantoin
(C) colchicine
(D) sulfamethoxazole
(E) phenylhydrazine

387. All the following statements concerning benign monoclonal gammopathy are true EXCEPT

(A) 10 to 20 percent of patients will develop multiple myeloma or other B-cell malignancy
(B) it is the result of proliferation of a single clone of B cells
(C) osteolysis does not occur
(D) the defect in humoral immunity leads to an increased incidence of infection with encapsulated organisms
(E) renal tubular dysfunction may occur secondary to light-chain excretion

DIRECTIONS: Each question below contains four suggested responses of which **one or more** is correct. Select

A	if	**1, 2, and 3**	are correct
B	if	**1 and 3**	are correct
C	if	**2 and 4**	are correct
D	if	**4**	is correct
E	if	**1, 2, 3, and 4**	are correct

388. True statements concerning prostate cancer and its treatment include that

(1) bone metastases are uniformly osteoblastic
(2) 95 percent are adenocarcinomas
(3) radiation therapy rarely causes impotence
(4) histologically, tumors are frequently multifocal

389. Introduction to general use of new chemotherapeutic drugs for cancer follows years of preclinical and clinical research. True statements regarding this research include which of the following?

(1) Phase II trials are undertaken only for drugs that have demonstrated encouraging activity in phase I studies
(2) Phase II trials are usually comparative studies with two or more treatment arms
(3) Phase III drugs are more active than phase I drugs
(4) Randomization of treatment assignment is used in phase III studies

390. Large cell non-Hodgkin's lymphoma and Hodgkin's disease are potentially curable diseases. Statements true of both diseases include

(1) 90 percent of cases are of B-cell origin
(2) curative chemotherapy requires multiple drugs
(3) gene rearrangement studies reveal clonality
(4) radiation may be curative in localized disease

391. Correct statements concerning drug-induced hemolytic anemia include that

(1) 10 percent of patients taking α-methyldopa will develop a Coombs-positive hemolytic anemia
(2) quinidine-induced hemolytic anemia is seen only during administration of high doses of the drug
(3) hemolytic anemia secondary to penicillin usually begins during the first 3 days of administration
(4) patients with a history of hemolytic anemia to penicillin have an increased likelihood of developing a hemolytic anemia to cephalosporins

392. A young woman presents with a small breast nodule, which on needle biopsy is found to be an adenocarcinoma. Examination is otherwise unremarkable and results of laboratory studies are normal. Interventions likely to be curative include

(1) radical mastectomy with full axillary dissection
(2) lumpectomy with axillary sampling followed by radiotherapy
(3) simple mastectomy without axillary dissection
(4) pulse chemotherapy and hormonal therapy without additional local treatment

393. A 20-year-old man is being investigated for severe normocytic normochromic anemia (hematocrit 28 percent). Mild granulocytopenia and thrombocytopenia are present. The patient is found to have hemosiderinuria but no hemoglobinuria. He has a low leukocyte alkaline phosphatase level and a low red blood cell acetylcholinesterase level. Management of this condition includes

(1) corticosteroid treatment
(2) washed red cell transfusions
(3) administration of heparin
(4) administration of fluoxymesterone, 20 to 30 mg/day

394. Adjuvant therapy is given to patients who no longer have detectable residual cancer following primary resection of disease but who are considered to be at risk for recurrence. The largest group of patients receiving adjuvant treatment are those with breast cancer. True statements regarding adjuvant treatment of breast cancer include

(1) disease-free survival is improved
(2) overall survival may be improved
(3) younger patients obtain more benefit from chemotherapy, but patients over 50 do better with hormonal treatment
(4) many patients are cured by adjuvant treatment

395. Cytogenetic abnormalities can now be detected in the majority of patients with acute myelogenous leukemia. True statements regarding these abnormalities include

(1) cytogenetic results correlate with morphology
(2) cytogenetic results predict treatment response
(3) cytogenetic findings resolve at remission
(4) cytogenetic results predict clinical course

DIRECTIONS: Each group of questions below consists of lettered headings followed by a set of numbered items. For each numbered item select the **one** lettered heading with which it is **most** closely associated. Each lettered heading may be used **once, more than once, or not at all.**

Questions 396–400

Match the following.

(A) Methotrexate
(B) Cytosine arabinoside
    (cytarabine)
(C) Nitrogen mustard
(D) Cyclophosphamide
(E) Doxorubicin

396.   A synthetic alkylating agent that must be activated by the mixed function oxidases in hepatic microsomes. Hydration and adequate urinary flow help to prevent cystitis resulting from this drug

397.   A synthetic alkylating agent that, being very reactive in aqueous solution, must be used within minutes of solubilization. It causes a severe chemical burn (cellulitis) if extravasation occurs

398.   A folic acid antagonist that is excreted by the kidneys essentially unchanged. Renal function must be assessed, therefore, prior to use. Chronic use may produce hepatic cirrhosis

399.   An antitumor antibiotic that is very useful in the treatment of the lymphomas, sarcomas, acute leukemia, and breast cancer. Dose-related cardiomyopathy limits the cumulative dose

400.   An antimetabolite particularly effective against acute leukemia. Dose-limiting effects include CNS, mucosal, and hepatic toxicities

Questions 401–405

Match the descriptions below with the appropriate pathologic inclusions.

(A) Howell-Jolly bodies
(B) Pappenheimer bodies
(C) Cabot rings (ring bodies)
(D) Heinz bodies
(E) Coarse basophilic stippling

401. Seen in splenectomized patients and in those with hemolytic anemia

402. Seen in megaloblastic anemia; origin unknown

403. Iron granulations

404. An intracellular precipitate of hemoglobin

405. Aggregated ribosomes; characteristic of lead intoxication and thalassemia

DIRECTIONS: Each group of questions below consists of four lettered headings followed by a set of numbered items. For each numbered item select

A	if the item is associated with	(A) **only**
B	if the item is associated with	(B) **only**
C	if the item is associated with	**both** (A) and (B)
D	if the item is associated with	**neither** (A) nor (B)

Each lettered heading may be used **once, more than once, or not at all.**

Questions 406–410

(A) Benign gastric ulcer
(B) Malignant gastric ulcer
(C) Both
(D) Neither

406. Affected patients may present with epigastric distress, easy fatigability, anemia, and guaiac-positive stools

407. Affected patients respond to antacid therapy both symptomatically and roentgenographically

408. Affected patients may be genetically predisposed

409. Differential diagnosis includes lymphoma, pseudolymphoma, and Ménétrier's disease

410. Disease may be associated with elevated carcinoembryonic antigen titers

Questions 411–415

(A) Hemophilia A (factor VIII coagulant deficiency)
(B) Hemophilia B (factor IX deficiency)
(C) Both
(D) Neither

411. Possible carrier detection by comparison of coagulant factor and the von Willebrand factor levels

412. Vitamin K–dependent protein

413. Prolonged template bleeding time

414. Response to cryoprecipitate

415. Response to desmopressin (DDAVP)

Questions 416–420

   (A) Iron deficiency
   (B) Anemia of chronic disease
   (C) Both
   (D) Neither

416.   Increased reticulocyte production

417.   Increased free erythrocyte protoporphyrin (FEP)

418.   Increased anisocytosis

419.   Decreased ratio of iron to total iron-binding capacity (TIBC)

420.   Exclusion by serum ferritin level of 100 μg/L

Questions 421–425

   (A) Chronic myelogenous leukemia (CML)
   (B) Agnogenic mycloid metaplasia (AMM)
   (C) Both
   (D) Neither

421.   Increase in the absolute basophil count

422.   Typically absent leukocyte alkaline phosphatase

423.   Philadelphia chromosome

424.   Osteosclerosis

425.   Tendency toward a chronic phase over many years

Questions 426–430

   (A) Thrombotic thrombocytopenic purpura (TTP)
   (B) Chronic idiopathic thrombocytopenic purpura (chronic ITP)
   (C) Both
   (D) Neither

426.   Normal or increased numbers of megakaryocytes

427.   Steroid therapy

428.   Fever

429.   Fragmented red cells

430.   Possible presence of serum antiplatelet antibodies

Questions 431–435

(A) Acute lymphocytic leukemia
    (ALL)
(B) Acute myelocytic leukemia
    (AML)
(C) Both
(D) Neither

431.   Most frequent in children and may be curable

432.   Usually fatal within 3 months if the affected patient is untreated or fails to respond to therapy

433.   Histochemical tests are useful in determining subtypes. Affected cells usually stain positively with peroxidase, Sudan black, and esterase stains

434.   Chromosomal abnormalities occur and are diagnostic

435.   Treatment typically renders affected patients severely hypoplastic or aplastic for a period of time, requiring intensive supportive care

Oncology and Hematology

Answers

378.   The answer is D. *(Williams, ed 4. pp 1362-1363, 1575-1576. Wilson, ed 12. pp 1511, 1512.)* Hemorrhage is the most frequent complication of heparin therapy and may occur even at optimal therapeutic levels. Heparin causes thrombocytopenia in up to 5 percent of patients and may be associated with diffuse platelet activation and thrombosis. Prompt diagnosis of heparin-associated thrombosis is crucial since continuation of heparin will lead to progressive thrombosis. Heparin use for periods in excess of 2 months may produce osteoporosis. Skin necrosis is associated with vitamin K–antagonist anticoagulation of patients with deficiency of protein C or S activity. In these patients the imbalance between vitamin K–dependent procoagulant and anticoagulant activity is exacerbated during the initial period of vitamin K antagonism, resulting in thrombosis. This complication can apparently be avoided by concurrent heparin administration during initial vitamin K antagonism.

379.   The answer is C. *(Wilson, ed 4. pp 209-211, 251-266, 994-1003, 1079-1081. Wilson, ed 12. pp 1553-1575.)* At least 50 percent of children with ALL are cured by current standard-dose therapy, while fewer adults are saved. Treatment of AML is less successful, but at least 25 percent of patients who achieve remission are long-term survivors. Approximately 75 percent of patients with high-grade lymphoma achieve initial remission and 50 percent of these appear to be cured. CML is only palliated by standard-dose therapies, which have little effect on survival. Cure is currently possible in CML only by marrow ablation and bone marrow transplantation.

380.   The answer is B. *(Williams, ed 4. pp 613-625. Wilson, ed 12. pp 1543-1545.)* Clinical laboratory testing is not useful in the diagnosis of a painful crisis. Hemoglobin, reticulocyte number, bilirubin, and lactic dehydrogenase levels, which are typically abnormal in patients with sickle cell disease, do not fluctuate during crisis. Splenic function is an early casualty of sickle cell disease, with most splenic function lost in childhood because of repeated thrombosis. Treatment for sickle cell crisis is supportive with intravenous fluids and pain control. Transfusion is not helpful in usual crisis, but may be useful for stroke in evolution or prevention of stroke recurrence. Chest and hepatic crisis may also respond. Aggressive transfusion during pregnancy may be useful in women with sickle cell disease and recurrent abortion.

381.   The answer is A. *(Wilson, ed 12. p 64.)* Oncogenes have been identified in *all* human and animal tissue studied. The identification of oncogenes may explain the long-observed relationship between various types of cancer and DNA damage, such as that from exposure to alkylating drugs or radiation. Such damage may result in altered oncogene regulation or expression. Similarly, insertion of viral oncogenes via retroviral vectors could produce malignancy. At least two types of retroviral oncoviruses have been identified. One type interferes with regulation of cellular proto-oncogenes, which results in malignancy usually after a long latent period. The second type of retrovirus serves as a vector for a viral oncogene, which may rapidly induce malignant transformation.

382.   The answer is B. *(Williams, ed 4. pp 453–481.)* Vitamin B_{12} deficiency is an important cause of megaloblastosis and develops in the vast majority of cases as a result of impaired vitamin B_{12} absorption. Normally vitamin B_{12} is bound to intrinsic factor (IF) secreted into the stomach, and vitamin B_{12} bound to IF is absorbed by ileal mucosa. This mechanism fails if the stomach does not secrete IF or if IF secreted is not available for vitamin B_{12} binding. The latter occurs in pernicious anemia, where an anti-IF antibody blocks vitamin B_{12} binding. Vitamin B_{12} can be stripped from IF by bacterial overgrowth that occurs in small-bowel diverticula or other blind loops. Diffuse ileal abnormality in Crohn's disease or sprue and, rarely, lymphoma or other processes may also result in deficiency, as can tapeworm infestation. The cause of deficiency should be sought since types of management differ. Detection of IF antibody is diagnostic of pernicious anemia but is found in only a minority of patients. A several-stage Schilling test is undertaken if IF antibody is negative, but only after a period of vitamin B_{12} replacement because megaloblastosis of the gut should be corrected prior to the Schilling test. Part I of the Schilling test measures urinary excretion of an oral dose of radiolabeled vitamin B_{12} administered after sufficient parenteral vitamin B_{12} is administered to saturate vitamin B_{12} binding sites so that additional vitamin B_{12} absorbed is excreted in urine. If excretion is low, the test is repeated (part II) with the addition of IF. If absorption in Schilling part II remains low, the test is repeated after a course of oral antibiotics. Bacterial overgrowth will result in abnormal excretion in both parts I and II of the Schilling and is corrected by antibiotics.

383.   The answer is D. *(Williams, ed 4. pp 158–167.)* Blood product support is essential in managing aplastic anemia but transfusion may be associated with alloimmunization and may impair engraftment. Transfusion should be minimized and transfusions from family members avoided if BMT is a consideration. Survival before effective therapies were developed was brief in most patients with severe aplastic anemia, as it is in those patients failing to respond to current treatment. Immunosuppressive therapy may be successful in severe aplastic anemia regardless of etiologic association, unless aplasia is due to bone marrow ablation. BMT is the treatment of choice for younger patients with severe aplastic anemia and for most patients with an identical twin. Toxicity of allogeneic but not isogeneic BMT remains age-related.

384.   The answer is B. *(Williams, ed 4. pp 546–548.)* Myelophthisic anemia is caused by marrow infiltration due most often to malignancy but also occurs as a result of infectious or inflammatory disorders involving the marrow and in metabolic storage disorders with deposition of lipid in marrow. Myelophthisic anemia varies widely in severity. It is characterized by disordered and premature release of cells from marrow or sites of extramedullary hematopoiesis. Teardrop-shaped red cells are typically seen along with myeloid precursors and nucleated red cells on the peripheral blood film as disease progresses. The diagnosis of myelophthisic anemia requires marrow examination, usually including marrow biopsy, since aspiration is often impossible and is otherwise less sensitive than biopsy in making the diagnosis. Treatment is directed toward the underlying disease where possible, transfusion support may be required by symptoms. Hypersplenism may respond to splenectomy in selected patients. Acanthocytes are seen in diseases that result in abnormal red cell lipid content, as occurs in severe hepatic disease or abetalipoproteinemia.

385.   The answer is D. *(Wilson, ed 12. pp 1563–1565.)* Polycythemia vera is a chronic progressive disease characterized by an increased production of myeloid elements and splenomegaly. In distinction to the secondary forms of polycythemia, urine and serum levels of erythropoietin are substantially reduced or absent. Red blood cell mass, hemoglobin concentration, hematocrit, and total blood volume are all elevated. Symptoms relating to the associated increased viscosity and reduced cerebral perfusion include headache, tinnitus, visual alterations, and stroke. Peripheral vascular symptoms are common and the incidence of peptic ulcer disease is increased. Early satiety and abdominal fullness are related to the associated splenomegaly. Bleeding is common. Laboratory findings include an elevated hemoglobin concentration, leukocytosis with an increase in the absolute basophil count, thrombocytosis, and a very low erythrocyte sedimentation rate. Bone marrow examination reveals a panmyelosis with absent or markedly reduced iron stores. Progression to marrow fibrosis occurs in up to 20 percent of patients. The majority of patients die of vascular complications. Acute leukemia develops in less than 5 percent of patients but risk is increased by chlorambucil and presumably other alkylating agents. The use of these drugs is now generally avoided since radioactive phosphorus or hydroxyurea can control marrow proliferation in patients who require more treatment than phlebotomy without the leukemia risk of chlorambucil. The goal of treatment is to reduce blood viscosity and thus restore perfusion by decreasing red cell mass, hemoglobin, and hematocrit to the normal range. Platelet count may rise markedly during phlebotomy and thrombocytosis may contribute to vascular events. Iron-deficient erythropoiesis is associated with stiff red cell membranes, which increase blood viscosity. The role of platelets and red cell membrane abnormalities in the pathogenesis of vascular complications of polycythemia rubra vera is poorly understood, but apparently is much less important than red cell mass. Antiplatelet agents increase hemorrhagic risk but have not demonstrated efficacy in preventing stroke and should not be used routinely.

386. The answer is C. *(Williams, ed 4. pp 598–599.)* Glucose-6-phosphate dehydrogenase (G6PD) deficiency is a hereditary disease characterized by a decreased activity of the enzyme and the consequent predisposition of red cells to hemolyze as a result of drugs, infection, or acidosis. Drug-induced hemolysis results from the complexing of oxidized glutathione to hemoglobin, which precipitates as Heinz bodies. Red cells containing these inclusions are rapidly removed from the circulation and hemolysis ensues. There are several types of G6PD deficiency and the severity of the drug-induced hemolytic anemia is different for each; furthermore, people with the same G6PD variant may exhibit different degrees of hemolysis to the same drug. Other than the drugs mentioned in the question—excluding colchicine—the medications to be avoided include pentaquine, primaquine, sulfanilamide, and nalidixic acid. Treatment of severe hemolysis includes blood transfusions, maintenance of good urine flow, and the administration of vitamin E.

387. The answer is D. *(Williams, ed 4. pp 1109–1113.)* Benign monoclonal gammopathy is the most common disorder of immunoglobulins and is due to the proliferation of a single B lymphocyte clone that reaches a steady-state of less than 1×10^{11} total cells. Bone destruction, marrow depression, and a susceptibility to infection are not seen. The syndrome is found incidentally. Laboratory values are unremarkable although a drop in alternative levels of immunoglobulin may occur. Marrow plasma cell concentration is normal. Most patients remain asymptomatic but up to 20 percent will eventually progress to multiple myeloma, macroglobulinemia, or B-cell lymphoma.

388. The answer is C (2, 4). *(Wilson, ed 12. pp 1630–1632.)* Prostate cancers, which are most commonly adenocarcinomas, are the second most common malignancy in men. They may spread by direct extension, hematogenously, or via the lymphatics, and commonly cause both osteoblastic and osteoclastic bone metastases. Staging is divided into four main groups with stages A and B designating tumor confined to the prostate and stages C and D tumor spread beyond the capsule. Treatment for cancer of the prostate involves surgery, radiation therapy, hormonal therapy, and chemotherapy in various combinations dependent on the type and stage of the tumor. In patients receiving external beam radiation, 30 to 60 percent suffer impotence.

389. The answer is D (4). *(Wilson, ed 12. pp 1590–1591.)* Chemotherapeutic drugs are examined for possible clinical use in a series of trials. In phase I studies, drugs that have shown promise in the laboratory are evaluated to determine the tolerable dose, schedule, and clinical pharmacokinetics of a given drug. Once optimal dose and schedule are defined, phase II studies evaluate clinical activity. If useful activity is suggested in phase II, comparison with standard regimens is evaluated in randomized phase III studies.

390.   The answer is C (2, 4). *(Williams, ed 4. pp 1031–1088. Wilson, ed 12. pp 1603–1612.)* The curative potential of multiple-agent chemotherapeutic regimens was first demonstrated in Hodgkin's disease, and the potential for cure with such treatment was subsequently shown in non-Hodgkin's lymphoma. Most cases of non-Hodgkin's lymphoma are of B-cell origin as established by surface phenotype or immunoglobulin gene rearrangement study. T-cell origin can be shown in a minority of patients on the basis of surface phenotype or T-cell receptor rearrangement. The cell of origin for Hodgkin's disease is unknown. Radiation is potentially curative in early-stage lymphoma of either Hodgkin's or non-Hodgkin's type.

391.   The answer is D (4). *(Williams, ed 4. pp 681–685.)* Three mechanisms explain the pathogenesis of drug-induced hemolytic anemia. In the immune complex mechanism characterized by quinidine, isoniazid, sulfonamides, and phenacetin, the drug combines with preformed antibody. The resultant complexes bind reversibly to red cells, which are then hemolyzed by fixed complement. Only small amounts of drug are needed for hemolysis because the immune complexes are capable of migrating from cell to cell. α-Methyldopa, in contrast, seems to cause a hemolytic anemia by inactivating suppressor-cell function, allowing autoantibodies to form against red cell antigens. Fully 10 percent of people taking α-methyldopa will be Coombs-positive but less than 1 percent will experience a hemolytic anemia, usually 3 to 6 months after initiating therapy. In hapten-mediated anemia, the involved drug coats circulating red cells and is then bound by specific antibody; the immune complex-coated erythrocytes are destroyed through splenic sequestration. Penicillin and the cephalosporins (which have antigenic cross-reactivity with penicillin) are prime examples of this type of hemolytic anemia, which begins after 7 to 10 days of drug use.

392.   The answer is A (1, 2, 3). *(Wilson, ed 12. pp 1613–1618.)* Local treatments appear equally efficacious in controlling disease in the breast. Node dissection provides staging information of prognostic significance, but is not therapeutic. Recurrence in node-positive women is at least three times more frequent than in women without axillary involvement. Risk of recurrence increases in direct relation to the number of nodes involved.

393.   The answer is C (2, 4). *(Wilson, ed 12. pp 1538–1539.)* The patient presented in the question suffers from paroxysmal nocturnal hemoglobinuria (PNH). Notwithstanding the name of the syndrome, hemoglobinuria is seldom gross and may occur only intermittently—in some affected patients no more than trace amounts may ever occur. Similarly, the anemia associated with this condition is variable, being profound in only a few patients. Many patients exhibit normal levels of hemoglobin or only moderate reductions. The diagnosis, however, would be extremely unlikely in the absence of hemosiderin in the urine. A preliminary diagnosis of PNH is confirmed with an acid hemolysis test or sucrose lysis test. Further confirmation would be evidence of low concentrations of leukocyte alkaline phosphatase and red blood cell acetylcholinesterase. Activation of the terminal part of the complement cascade normally is associated with some red blood cell lysis. However, patients with PNH are inordinately sensitive to these complement components. In addition to erythrocytes, granulocytes and platelets also are sensitive to these mechanisms. Transfusions of packed red cells or washed packed red cells are usually beneficial. Although blood transfusions contain complement components and their substrates, this potential danger is offset by the passive increase in hemoglobin levels that follows transfusion. The increase in hemoglobin will suppress bone marrow production of young erythrocytes, which are particularly sensitive to complement. For similar reasons, the administration of ferrous sulfate to promote increased erythropoiesis will lead to the production of excessive numbers of young erythrocytes that will be destroyed by complement. Therapy with androgens, such as fluoxymesterone, frequently decreases the destruction of red blood cells and allows hemoglobin levels to rise. Steroids have been shown to affect both complement and red blood cells; however, their mechanism of action in this disease is not certain. PNH frequently is complicated by venous thromboses, for which prophylactic anticoagulation will be necessary. Coumarin-type drugs are useful in such situations, but heparin, which has been found actually to increase the rate of hemolysis, should be avoided.

394.   The answer is A (1, 2, 3). *(Wilson, ed 12. pp 1618–1619.)* The major benefit of current adjuvant treatment in breast cancer appears to be an increase in disease-free survival; it has less impact on overall survival. There is no clear evidence to recommend current treatment as curative. The role of adjuvant treatment in node-negative patients remains unresolved. Since many of these patients will not develop recurrent disease after primary treatment, a major advantage would have to be conferred on the subset of patients who would otherwise have recurrence to justify the cost and toxicity of treatment in the entire group. It is conceivable, however, that a more limited occult disease burden, in node-negative as compared with node-positive patients, may permit greater success with adjuvant treatment in node-negative patients. Additional studies will be required to resolve these issues.

395.   The answer is E (all). *(Wilson, ed 12. pp 1553–1559.)* There is a close association between specific morphologic subtypes of leukemia and cytogenetic abnormalities. Promyelocytic leukemia, t(15;17); myelomonocytic leukemia with eosinophilia, inv 16; and monocytic leukemia, t(9;11) are good examples in which there are distinctive morphologic and cytogenetic findings as well as characteristic clinical complications, such as disseminated intravascular coagulation in t(15;17) and skin, meningeal, and mucosal infiltration in t(9;11). Treatment prospects vary widely between leukemic subsets and indicate a need to explore different treatment strategies in various subgroups. Cytogenetic abnormalities are no longer found at remission with standard techniques, but more sensitive cytogenetic probes are being studied for possible use in monitoring remission status.

396–400.   The answers are: 396-D, 397-C, 398-A, 399-E, 400-B. *(Wilson, ed 12. pp 1587–1593.)* Cyclophosphamide is a broadly active alkylating agent useful in hematologic and solid tumor neoplasia. It is metabolized to its active form by liver microsomes. Acrolein is a reactive metabolite of cyclophosphamide that is excreted in urine and may cause hemorrhagic cystitis. This risk can be minimized by maintaining a dilute urine and by frequent voiding.

Nitrogen mustard was the first effective chemotherapeutic agent developed. Its major use is in the treatment of Hodgkin's disease. Toxic manifestations other than those listed in the question include nausea, vomiting, bone marrow suppression, and alopecia.

Methotrexate was designed and functions as a folate antagonist. Drug development was encouraged by the observation that exogenous folic acid appeared to accelerate the progression of acute leukemia. Methotrexate has broad activity, including activity against acute leukemia, breast cancer, head and neck cancer, choriocarcinoma, and sarcoma. Major dose-limiting effects of methotrexate include renal and mucosal toxicity as well as bone marrow suppression. Cumulative hepatic toxicity may develop.

Doxorubicin is isolated from *Streptomyces peucetius*. It functions as an inhibitor of DNA synthesis via intercalation into the DNA molecule. Side effects other than cardiotoxicity include nausea, vomiting, bone marrow suppression, alopecia, and mucositis. It is a potent vesicant if extravasated.

Cytosine arabinoside (also called cytarabine and Ara-C) is an analogue of the naturally occurring cytosine ribonucleoside. Ara-C is activated via cytidine kinase to the active nucleotide Ara-CTP, which competes with CTP for the polymerase enzyme. It is particularly effective against acute leukemia. CNS, mucosal, and hepatic toxicities are dose-limiting. Because of its short half-life, and since Ara-C activity is limited to cycling cells, it is given in repeated injections or as a constant infusion. Oral Ara-C is ineffective because the high concentration of cytidine deaminase in the intestinal mucosa converts Ara-C to the inactive uracil arabinoside.

401–405.   The answers are: 401-A, 402-C, 403-B, 404-D, 405-E. *(Williams, ed 4. p 308.)* Pathologic inclusions are nuclear or cytoplasmic remnants that are present in various disease states. Howell-Jolly bodies are nuclear remnants that are either chromosomes that have separated from the mitotic spindle during mitosis (the result of nuclear fragmentation) or the product of incomplete nuclear expulsion. They are normally removed during passage through the spleen. Howell-Jolly bodies are found in patients with hemolytic anemia or megaloblastic anemia, and in those who have been splenectomized.

Cabot rings (ring bodies), which usually appear as singular rings in reticulocytes on Wright's-stained film, are found in megaloblastic anemias; their origin is unknown.

Pappenheimer bodies are peripherally located siderosomes and appear as small, dense blue granules on Wright's stain.

Heinz bodies are found in patients with hemoglobin variants. Because of their decreased solubility, these abnormal hemoglobins readily precipitate. Red cells with Heinz bodies are removed by the reticuloendothelial system.

Basophilic stippling occurs in conditions of abnormal hemoglobin biosynthesis and represents aggregates of ribosomes. It is a characteristic feature of lead intoxication and thalassemias.

406–410.   The answers are: 406-C, 407-C, 408-B, 409-B, 410-B. *(Wilson, ed 12. pp 1229–1241.)* The clinical histories associated with benign and malignant gastric ulcers tend to be quite similar. The peak incidence for benign ulcer disease is between 45 and 55 years of age; for gastric carcinoma, it is 55 years of age. Both benign and malignant ulcer diseases affect men more frequently than women, the ratio being 3.5:1 for the benign disease and 2:1 for the malignant. While benign gastric ulcer disease does not appear to have a familial predisposition, gastric cancer is two to four times more common in relatives of affected patients than in the general population.

Symptoms of benign gastric ulcers may be quite vague; easy satiety and nausea after eating are common complaints. Midepigastric pain may be aggravated by eating, and weight loss is frequent. Bleeding results in guaiac-positive stools, and secondary anemia and weight loss result in easy fatigability.

Although the clinical history associated with benign gastric ulcers is shared by the majority of patients afflicted with malignant gastric ulcers, approximately 25 percent of such patients present classic *duodenal* ulcer symptoms, including midepigastric burning pain relieved by food.

Preoperative differentiation between benign and malignant ulcer disease is possible in 80 to 90 percent of cases. Radiology can accurately differentiate between them approximately 85 percent of the time. Gastroscopy, cytologic examination, and biopsy of the lesions yield a diagnostic accuracy as high as 90 percent. False positive cytologic results are exceedingly uncommon; most diagnostic errors arise from false negatives. Examination of gastric acid is very helpful; true achlorhydria following maximal pentagastric stimulation excludes a benign gastric ulcer.

The presence of acid does not rule out gastric carcinoma. Moreover, improvement in response to medical therapy, both subjectively and on x-ray, can occur in patients who have malignant ulcers. If, following testing, doubt persists as to whether or not the lesion is benign, the affected patient should have surgery.

Conditions that may mimic malignant ulcers on x-ray include peptic ulcer disease, hypertrophic pyloric stenosis, antral gastritis, inflammatory polyps, Ménétrier's disease, lymphoma, pseudolymphoma, Crohn's disease, gastric varices, hematoma, and bezoars or retained food. Unfortunately, carcinoembryonic antigen (CEA) levels are elevated in most patients only after cancer has metastasized and thus the CEA measurement is not useful in early detection. Serial CEA measurements may be useful in evaluating response to treatment.

411–415. The answers are: 411-A, 412-D, 413-D, 414-A, 415-A. *(Williams, ed 4. pp 1449–1471. Wilson, ed 12. pp 1505–1507.)* The von Willebrand factor serves a carrier protein function for factor VIII coagulant, and levels of the two proteins are similar in normal persons and those with hemophilia B but divergent in patients with and most carriers of hemophilia A. Assays of factor VIII activity and antigen will likewise be linked except in hemophilia A variants in which a functionally deficient but antigenically reactive molecule is produced. Neither factor VIII nor factor IX is measured in the bleeding time, which is normal in both hemophilia A and B. A markedly prolonged bleeding time in a patient with low factor VIII coagulant levels is typical of von Willebrand's disease. Cryoprecipitate contains primarily fibrinogen, the von Willebrand factor, and factor VIII. DDAVP enhances endothelial release of the von Willebrand factor and with it factor VIII coagulant protein.

416–420. The answers are: 416-D, 417-C, 418-A, 419-C, 420-D. *(Williams, ed 4. pp 482–506, 540–546. Wilson, ed 12. pp 1519–1521.)* The primary aspect of both iron deficiency and anemia of chronic disease is inadequate synthesis of red cells. Reticulocytes are decreased. FEP levels are increased in both iron deficiency and anemia of chronic disease. Variation in cell size (anisocytosis) is a characteristic finding in iron deficiency but not in anemia of chronic disease. Serum iron may be extremely low in both disorders and has no discriminant value. If TIBC is elevated in association with a low serum iron, the diagnosis of iron deficiency is established. Ferritin levels between 10 and 90 are not diagnostic.

421–425. The answers are: 421-C, 422-A, 423-A, 424-B, 425-B. *(Wilson, ed 12. pp 1561–1563, 1565–1566.)* Both CML and AMM represent neoplasms of multipotent hematopoietic stem cells. CML is characterized by splenomegaly and increased numbers of granulocytes, particularly neutrophils; the white blood cell count often exceeds 200,000/mm³. Presenting symptoms are related to splenomegaly, anemia, or hypermetabolism; arthralgias, thrombohemorrhagic complications, and, rarely, lymphadenopathy are also seen. CML generally runs a mild course until it transforms into an accelerated or blastic phase, when the marrow produces

186 Medicine

increased numbers of blasts and promyelocytes. Laboratory findings include a marked leukocytosis, basophilia, elevated serum B_{12} levels, markedly reduced or absent leukocyte alkaline phosphatase levels, and hyperuricemia. More than 95 percent of patients have the Philadelphia chromosome, which consists of a reciprocal translocation of genetic material between the long arms of chromosome 22 and chromosome 9 with fusion of the c-*abl* oncogene from chromosome 9 with DNA from a specific region of chromosome 22 called the breakpoint cluster region. This results in synthesis of a chimeric protein that may be of importance in the pathophysiology of CML. AMM has no characteristic cytogenetic association. Laboratory findings and clinical course are more variable in AMM than in CML. Many AMM patients remain stable for years without treatment.

426–430.   The answers are: 426-C, 427-C, 428-A, 429-A, 430-B. *(Williams, ed 4. pp 1355–1359, 1378–1380.)* TTP is characterized by microangiopathic hemolytic anemia, thrombocytopenia, and neurologic dysfunction with the variable presence of fever and renal disease. The disorder may be either chronic or, more commonly, acute. Patients present with fluctuating neurologic abnormalities such as seizures, mental status changes, behavioral disorders, jaundice, purpura, and various manifestations of diffuse microinfarction, such as abdominal pain and complete heart block,- caused by widespread hyaline occlusions of small vessels. The peripheral smear is consistent with microangiopathic hemolytic anemia; thrombocytopenia, hyperbilirubinemia, leukocytosis, proteinuria, and hematuria are other frequent findings. Therapy involves a combination of glucocorticoids and plasma infusion or plasma exchange or both. Platelet inhibitors may be useful in some patients. Remission is achieved in 60 to 80 percent of cases but relapse may occur.

Chronic ITP, in contrast, is characterized by thrombocytopenia due to well-characterized immune-mediated mechanisms. The disease begins insidiously; patients present with cutaneous and mucosal bleeding. Thrombocytopenia is typically isolated, with normal RBC and WBC levels, unless there has been severe bleeding or in the rare patient who presents with both ITP and Coombs-positive hemolysis. Platelet-associated IgG is elevated. Ten to twenty percent of patients recover spontaneously. Treatment includes steroids to suppress the reticuloendothelial uptake of antibody-coated platelets. Patients who fail to respond to steroids or require high-dose steroid therapy to maintain an adequate platelet count are considered for additional treatment. Splenectomy is effective in increasing platelet count in more than 70 percent of patients and response is usually durable. ITP is more common in women and some patients will respond to the male hormone danazol; although the mechanism of action is unclear, responses are seen in both men and women. High-dose intravenous gamma globulin is also effective but only for brief periods—presumably by blocking reticuloendothelial Fc receptors. Vincristine and, to a lesser extent, azathioprine and other cytotoxic drugs have limited activity in resistant patients. ITP may be more common during pregnancy and transplacental transfer of antiplatelet antibody may cause fetal/neonatal thrombocytopenia with a risk of CNS bleeding at delivery. Pathophysiologic mechanisms of TTP are less well defined.

431–435. The answers are: 431-A, 432-C, 433-B, 434-C, 435-C. *(Wilson, ed 12. pp 1552–1559.)* The peak incidence of acute lymphocytic leukemia (ALL) is between the ages of 2 and 4 years. Although ALL also occurs in adults, adult leukemia is predominantly myelogenous. The sexes are equally affected in very young children; however, in older patients, ALL shows a slight male predominance (3:2).

Patients with all types of acute leukemia who fail to respond to therapy have a median survival of approximately 3 months. Death usually results from one of the complications of bone marrow failure, i.e., infection or bleeding or both. However, current therapy allows 90 to 95 percent of children who have ALL to enter remission; the median survival is approximately 5 years. It is projected that 50 percent of these patients may be cured. Acute leukemia therapy is divided into several stages: induction, consolidation, central nervous system prophylaxis, and maintenance. Although approximately 50 to 70 percent of patients who have acute myelocytic leukemia (AML) will enter complete remission, the median duration of remissions is only 10 to 12 months.

It is important to distinguish the two major forms of acute leukemia because the therapy and prognosis in each are quite different. This differentiation can frequently be accomplished by the examination of Wright-stained smears of peripheral blood and bone marrow. In ALL, the lymphoblasts have a high nuclear:cytoplasmic ratio, scant nucleoli (one or two), and no Auer rods, and the myeloid elements that are present appear normal. The lymphoblasts stain positively with para-aminosalicylic acid (PAS) and negatively with peroxidase and Sudan black. In contrast, leukemic myeloblasts contain more nucleoli (two to four) in a homogeneous "ground glass" nucleus. Auer rods may be evident in the cytoplasm and other more mature myeloid elements may be abnormal. The myeloblasts stain positively with peroxidase and Sudan black.

Chromosomal abnormalities are common in both ALL and AML, and routine cytogenetic analysis is warranted for both diagnostic and prognostic purposes. Most carefully studied patients who have AML exhibit some chromosomal abnormality in number or structure or both.

Induction of remission produces profound cytopenia in both AML and ALL. Older induction regimens for ALL were less marrow-toxic but were also less successful.

Neurology

DIRECTIONS: Each question below contains five suggested responses. Select the **one best** response to each question.

436. A 45-year-old woman presents to her physician with an 8-month history of gradually increasing limb weakness. She first noticed difficulty climbing stairs, then problems rising from chairs, walking more than half a block, and, finally, lifting her arms above shoulder level. Aside from some difficulty swallowing, she has no ocular, bulbar, or sphincter problems, and no sensory complaints. Family history is negative for neurologic disease. Examination reveals significant proximal limb and neck muscle weakness with minimal atrophy, normal sensory findings, and intact deep tendon reflexes. The most likely diagnosis in this patient is

(A) polymyositis
(B) cervical myelopathy
(C) myasthenia gravis
(D) mononeuropathy multiplex
(E) limb girdle muscular dystrophy

437. A 55-year-old diabetic woman suddenly develops weakness of the left side of her face as well as of her right arm and leg. She also has diplopia on left lateral gaze. The lesion affecting this patient is probably located in the

(A) right cerebral hemisphere
(B) left cerebral hemisphere
(C) right side of the brainstem
(D) left side of the brainstem
(E) right medial longitudinal fasciculus

438. All the following are recognized neurologic complications of HIV (human immunodeficiency virus) infection EXCEPT

(A) dementia
(B) cerebral toxoplasmosis
(C) CNS astrocytoma
(D) myelopathy
(E) chronic inflammatory polyneuropathy

439. All the following statements concerning brain abscess are true EXCEPT

(A) common etiologic organisms include streptococci and *Escherichia coli*
(B) lumbar puncture is contraindicated in patients with a suspected brain abscess
(C) congenital heart disease is a common cause in children
(D) more than 50 percent of cases are due to skull fracture or intracranial surgery
(E) it is characterized by a ring-enhancing lesion on CT scan

440. A 19-year-old man tells his physician that he has been troubled for 4 days by a severe pain across the top of his right shoulder and the upper part of his right arm. He thought he might have injured the arm but became alarmed when the pain subsided and a progressive weakness developed. All the following comments related to this medical history would be reasonable EXCEPT

(A) he may well have received a tetanus toxoid shot in the arm a week before the pain started
(B) the patient is likely to have leukocytosis and an increased sedimentation rate
(C) EMG and nerve conduction studies may identify a local brachial plexus disturbance
(D) recovery of arm strength may take a year or longer
(E) the serratus anterior or deltoid muscles are more likely to be involved than the extensor carpi radialis and interosseous muscles

441. All the following statements about the treatment of Parkinson's disease are correct EXCEPT

(A) levodopa is usually administered in conjunction with carbidopa
(B) limb and facial dyskinesias are the most common side effects of chronic levodopa therapy
(C) levodopa treatment, while ameliorating symptoms, does not alter the natural history of the disease
(D) bromocriptine works by increasing the release of dopamine from the substantia nigra
(E) use of trihexyphenidyl and benztropine mesylate frequently causes confusional states and hallucinations

442. A patient arrives at a hospital breathing and with reactive pupils, but without other evidence of brain function. An electroencephalogram (EEG) shows electrocerebral silence (i.e., no cerebral activity). A reasonably good chance of full recovery exists if the underlying factor is

(A) cardiac arrest
(B) intracerebral hemorrhage
(C) encephalitis
(D) head trauma
(E) barbiturate overdose

443. Which of the following symptoms would suggest that the headaches suffered by a patient were due to migraine?

(A) Numbness or tingling of the left face, lips, and hand lasting for 5 to 15 min, followed by a throbbing headache
(B) An increasingly throbbing headache associated with unilateral visual loss and generalized muscle aching
(C) A continuous aching headache associated with sleepiness, nausea, ataxia, and incoordination of the right upper limb
(D) An intense left retroorbital headache associated with transient left-sided ptosis and rhinorrhea
(E) A visual field defect that persists following cessation of a unilateral headache

444. Diffuse hyperreflexia in a limb that is markedly atrophic and weak can be seen in which of the following disorders?

(A) Brachial plexus neuropathy involving the upper trunk
(B) Recent cerebral infarction with hemiparesis
(C) Cervical radiculopathy
(D) Multiple sclerosis
(E) Amyotrophic lateral sclerosis

445. A 45-year-old man with a history of heavy drinking is admitted to a hospital with diplopia, mild drowsiness, disorientation, and ataxia of a week's duration. On examination, the patient is found to be inattentive and unable to concentrate. He is disoriented to time and place and periodically falls asleep during conversation. He exhibits horizontal and vertical nystagmus and bilateral gaze palsies. Examination of the limbs reveals a symmetrical polyneuropathy. This diagnostic picture is most consistent with which of the following?

(A) Korsakoff's psychosis
(B) Marchiafava-Bignami disease
(C) Wernicke's disease
(D) Wernicke-Korsakoff syndrome
(E) Alcoholic cerebellar degeneration

446. A diagnosis of brain death requires all the following clinical signs EXCEPT

(A) irreversible cessation of respiration
(B) irreversible cessation of cardiac function
(C) pupils that are unreactive
(D) lack of response to oculocephalic testing
(E) lack of decerebrate posturing

DIRECTIONS: Each question below contains four suggested responses of which **one or more** is correct. Select

A	if	**1, 2, and 3**	are correct
B	if	**1 and 3**	are correct
C	if	**2 and 4**	are correct
D	if	**4**	is correct
E	if	**1, 2, 3, and 4**	are correct

447. A patient suffering from narcolepsy is likely to

(1) show early-onset REM (rapid eye movement) sleep after falling asleep
(2) experience terrifying hallucinations while falling asleep
(3) fall asleep while eating, standing, or driving
(4) have attacks of muscle paralysis stimulated by emotional or exciting experiences

448. Segmental demyelination is the primary pathologic process in which of the following subacute or chronic polyneuropathies?

(1) Isoniazid (INH) neuropathy
(2) Carcinomatous (paraneoplastic) polyneuropathy
(3) Alcoholic (nutritional) polyneuropathy
(4) Chronic inflammatory polyradiculoneuropathy

449. A middle-aged woman presenting with bilateral facial nerve palsy should be evaluated for which of the following diseases?

(1) Sarcoidosis
(2) Acute hepatitis
(3) Lyme disease
(4) Hypoparathyroidism

450. True statements concerning transient ischemic attacks (TIAs) include which of the following?

(1) TIAs are a predictor of cerebral and myocardial infarctions
(2) There are definite clinical features that indicate which patients with TIAs will develop a stroke
(3) Diplopia, bifacial numbness, and dysarthria imply vertebrobasilar disease
(4) TIAs of the carotid system commonly involve the eye and brain simultaneously

451. Correct statements concerning trauma-induced seizures include which of the following?

(1) Petit mal seizures occur commonly after trauma
(2) Most are controlled by anticonvulsant medication
(3) The greater the interval between injury and the first seizure, the more likely a complete remission will occur
(4) In the absence of a brain contusion or laceration, trauma does not increase the risk of developing seizures

SUMMARY OF DIRECTIONS

A	B	C	D	E
1, 2, 3 only	1, 3 only	2, 4 only	4 only	All are correct

452. True statements concerning pseudotumor cerebri include which of the following?

(1) Visual field testing commonly shows enlargement of the blind spots
(2) Mentation and alertness are often impaired
(3) It is most commonly found in young, obese women
(4) The most feared complication is brain herniation related to increased intracranial pressure

453. Correct statements concerning Huntington's chorea include which of the following?

(1) It is a hereditary disease with an autosomal dominant pattern
(2) There is a high association with chronic subdural hematoma
(3) Wasting of the head of the caudate nucleus and putamen is seen
(4) Choreoathetosis invariably precedes the manifestations of the psychic disorder

454. In a patient complaining of low back pain radiating down the right leg, which of the following clinical points would suggest a lesion compressing the first sacral root?

(1) Absent ankle reflex
(2) Pain in posterior thigh, posterior calf, and outer plantar surface of foot
(3) Diminished sensation in fourth and fifth toes
(4) Difficulty walking on heel

455. A 65-year-old man with recent onset of Broca's aphasia would likely have which of the following abnormalities on neurologic examination?

(1) Decrease in word output
(2) Difficulty repeating spoken words
(3) Weakness of the right face and arm
(4) Severe impairment in writing

456. A person sustaining an injury to the upper trunk of the brachial plexus is most likely to show weakness in which of the following muscles?

(1) Deltoid
(2) Triceps
(3) Infraspinatus
(4) Flexor carpi ulnaris

457. Correct statements concerning multiple sclerosis include which of the following?

(1) An attack of optic neuritis is generally required before the diagnosis can be made
(2) Seizures occur in approximately 50 percent of patients over the course of the disease
(3) Peripheral nerve involvement may be the initial manifestation
(4) Cerebellar ataxia may be found combined with sensory ataxia

458. Conditions due to remote effects of neoplasia on the nervous system (paraneoplastic disorders) include

(1) subacute combined degeneration
(2) cerebellar degeneration
(3) Creutzfeldt-Jakob disease
(4) Lambert-Eaton myasthenic syndrome

DIRECTIONS: Each group of questions below consists of lettered headings followed by a set of numbered items. For each numbered item select the **one** lettered heading with which it is **most** closely associated. Each lettered heading may be used **once, more than once, or not at all.**

Questions 459–463

Match each description to the appropriate tumor.

  (A) Meningioma
  (B) Astrocytoma
  (C) Glioblastoma multiforme
  (D) Hemangioblastoma
  (E) Medulloblastoma

459. Tendency to form large cavities; 50 percent of patients present with focal or generalized seizures; slowly growing with headache and other mental symptoms often present for many years before diagnosis

460. Sharply demarcated from brain tissue; psammoma bodies present microscopically; highest incidence in seventh decade; readily visualized by contrast-enhanced CT scan

461. Frequently fills the fourth ventricle; majority of patients are children 4 to 8 years of age; stumbling gait, frequent falls, and papilledema found on presentation

462. Accounts for 20 percent of all intracranial tumors; often bilateral or in more than one lobe of a hemisphere; may form distant foci on spinal roots; cerebral symptoms diffuse with seizures present in 30 to 40 percent of patients

463. Presents with dizziness, ataxia of gait, and symptoms and signs of increased intracranial pressure; polycythemia may be present; often displays dominant inheritance

Questions 464–467

Match each description below with the appropriate dementia-causing disorder.

(A) Hypothyroid dementia
(B) Normal pressure hydrocephalus
(C) Multi-infarct dementia
(D) Creutzfeldt-Jakob disease
(E) Alzheimer's disease

464. Aphasia, agnosia, and apraxia are common; memory loss prominent; familial occurrence well documented; silver-staining neuritic plaques seen throughout cortex

465. Stuttering course; often associated with distinct focal neurologic events; pseudobulbar palsy common; hypertension often present

466. Rapid progression; myoclonic jerks; distinctive EEG pattern; occurrence in those receiving injections of human growth hormone

467. Unsteadiness of gait with impairment of balance; urinary incontinence; may follow subarachnoid hemorrhage; CT scan important for diagnosis

DIRECTIONS: Each group of questions below consists of four lettered headings followed by a set of numbered items. For each numbered item select

A	if the item is associated with	(A) **only**
B	if the item is associated with	(B) **only**
C	if the item is associated with	**both** (A) and (B)
D	if the item is associated with	**neither** (A) nor (B)

Each lettered heading may be used **once, more than once, or not at all.**

Questions 468–471

(A) Absence (petit mal) seizures
(B) Complex partial seizures
(C) Both
(D) Neither

468. Postictal confusion

469. Automatisms

470. Three-per-second spike and wave discharges

471. Déjà vu experiences

Questions 472–475

(A) Guillain-Barré syndrome
(B) Myasthenia gravis
(C) Both
(D) Neither

472. Ocular and facial muscle involvement

473. Response to edrophonium

474. Respiratory insufficiency

475. Areflexia

Neurology

Answers

436.   The answer is A. *(Adams, ed 4. pp 1106–1109.)* Polymyositis is an acquired myopathy characterized by subacute symmetric weakness of proximal limb and trunk muscles that progresses over several weeks or months. When a characteristic skin rash occurs, the disease is known as dermatomyositis. In addition to progressive proximal limb weakness, the patient often presents with dysphagia and neck muscle weakness. Up to one-half of cases with polymyositis-dermatomyositis may have, in addition, features of connective tissue diseases (rheumatoid arthritis, lupus erythematosus, scleroderma, Sjögren's syndrome). Laboratory findings include an elevated serum CK level, an EMG showing myopathic potentials with fibrillations, and a muscle biopsy showing necrotic muscle fibers and inflammatory infiltrates. Polymyositis is clinically distinguished from the muscular dystrophies by its less prolonged course and lack of family history. It is distinguished from myasthenia gravis by its lack of ocular muscle involvement, absence of variability in strength over hours or days, and lack of response to anticholinesterase inhibitor drugs.

437.   The answer is D. *(Adams, ed 4. pp 636–640, 1808.)* This patient has weakness of the left face and the contralateral (right) arm and leg, commonly called a "crossed hemiplegia." Such crossed syndromes are characteristic of brainstem lesions. In this case the lesion is an infarct localized to the left inferior pons and caused by occlusion of a branch of the basilar artery. The infarct has damaged the left sixth and seventh cranial nerves in the left pons, resulting in the diplopia on left lateral gaze and the left facial weakness. Also damaged in the left pons is the left corticospinal tract, proximal to its decussation in the medulla; this damage causes weakness in the right arm and leg. This classic presentation has been called the Millard-Gubler syndrome.

438.   The answer is C. *(Adams, ed 4. pp 612–614.)* Neurologic complications of AIDS are either due to primary infection with the AIDS virus (HIV) or secondary to immunosuppression and occur in at least one-third of patients with AIDS. A common occurrence in later stages is the AIDS dementia complex, a progressive dementia associated with motor abnormalities and felt to be due to direct infection with HIV. Other CNS complications related to immunosuppression include cerebral toxoplasmosis, primary CNS lymphoma, and herpes simplex or zoster encephalitis. A myelopathy with vacuolar degeneration is common, and a variety of neuropathic conditions have been described, including a distal sensory polyneuropathy and both acute and chronic inflammatory demyelinating polyneuropathy.

439. The answer is D. *(Adams, ed 4. pp 556-570.)* Brain abscess is a focal suppurative cerebral inflammatory process with a mortality of 15 to 20 percent. Common predisposing factors include a contiguous source of infection (paranasal sinuses, middle ear), suppurative pulmonary infections (e.g., lung abscess), and cardiac abnormalities (e.g., congenital heart defects). Only about 10 percent of cases are secondary to infections brought from the outside (compound skull fractures, intracranial operations). The most common organisms depend on the source of the abscess and include anaerobic streptococci, *Bacteroides*, Enterobacteriaceae (*E. coli*, *Proteus*), staphylococci, and fungi (*Candida*). Patients usually present with various combinations of headache, drowsiness and confusion, focal or generalized seizures, and focal neurologic deficit. Because CSF findings are nonspecific and the risk of herniation is significant, lumbar puncture is contraindicated and CT scanning remains the diagnostic procedure of choice.

440. The answer is B. *(Adams, ed 4. pp 1065-1066.)* Local weakness involving one or both arms that begins with severe pain and progresses to weakness as the pain abates may indicate a brachial plexus neuropathy. Although this syndrome can develop without any precipitating cause being recognized, it is not uncommon for it to follow administration of immunization or viral infection. The upper part of the brachial plexus is usually involved, and thus the most commonly involved muscles are in the shoulder region (serratus anterior, supraspinatus, infraspinatus, deltoid). Sensory loss is usually minimal. EMG and nerve conduction studies usually identify a local nerve disturbance and myelography is generally not necessary. The prognosis is excellent and no specific treatment is required, though patients must be warned that sometimes it may take up to 2 years for a full return to normal function.

441. The answer is D. *(Adams, ed 4. pp 59, 937-943.)* Parkinson's disease (PD) is marked by depletion of dopamine-rich cells in the substantia nigra. The resulting decrease in striatal dopamine is the basis for the classic symptoms of rigidity, bradykinesia, and tremor. By far the most widely used treatment for PD has been the drug levodopa. Levodopa is converted to dopamine in the substantia nigra and then transported to the striatum, where it stimulates dopamine receptors. This is the basis for the drug's clinical effect on PD. Levodopa is usually administered with carbidopa (a decarboxylase inhibitor), thus preventing levodopa's destruction in the blood and allowing it to be given at a dose that is lower and less likely to cause nausea and vomiting. The major problems with levodopa have been (1) significant limb and facial dyskinesias in most cases on chronic therapy and (2) the fact that levodopa only treats PD symptomatically, with the disease process of neuronal loss in the substantia nigra continuing despite drug treatment. Other drugs can be used in the treatment of PD. Anticholinergic agents, such as trihexyphenidyl (Artane) and benztropine mesylate (Cogentin), work by restoring the balance between striatal dopamine and acetylcholine. They can have significant anticholinergic effects on the CNS, including confusional states and hallucinations. Bromocriptine and pergolide are dopamine agonists that work directly by stimulating dopamine receptors in the striatum; side effects of these drugs are similar to those of levodopa.

442.   The answer is E. *(Adams, ed 4. pp 285-286, 895-897.)* Patients in coma following sedative-hypnotic drug intoxication have a fairly good chance of full recovery, provided they are still breathing by the time help is available. Barbiturate overdose is one instance in which an EEG showing electrocerebral silence does not indicate brain death; rather, the depressant effects on the brain can be completely reversed. Extreme hypothermia, especially in combination with a mild intoxication, may also cause a comatose condition that is fully reversible.

443.   The answer is A. *(Adams, ed 4. pp 138-149.)* The differential diagnosis of headaches associated with neurologic or visual dysfunction is important because it encompasses a variety of disorders, some quite serious and others relatively benign. Classic (or neurologic) migraine is generally a familial disorder that begins in childhood or early adult life. Typically the onset of an episode is marked by the progression of a neurologic disturbance over 5 to 15 min, followed by a unilateral (or occasionally bilateral) throbbing headache lasting for several hours up to a day. The most common neurologic disturbance involves formed or unformed flashes of light that impair vision in one of the visual fields ("scintillating scotoma"). Other possible neurologic symptoms include numbness and tingling of the unilateral face, lips, and hand; weakness of an arm or leg; mild aphasia; and mental confusion. The transience of the neurologic symptoms distinguishes migraine from other more serious conditions that cause headaches. Persistence of a visual field defect, speech disturbance, or mild hemiparesis suggests a focal lesion (e.g., arteriovenous malformation with hemorrhage or infarct). In the case of persistent ataxia, limb incoordination, and nausea, one should consider a posterior fossa (possibly cerebellar) mass lesion. Monocular visual loss in an elderly patient with throbbing headaches should initiate a search for cranial (temporal) arteritis. This should include a sedimentation rate (usually elevated) and a temporal artery biopsy (which would show a giant cell arteritis). Fifty percent of these patients have the generalized muscle aching seen with polymyalgia rheumatica. Unilateral orbital or retroorbital headaches, occurring nightly for a period of 2 to 8 weeks, are characteristic of cluster headaches. These headaches are often associated with ipsilateral injection of the conjunctivum, nasal stuffiness, rhinorrhea, and, less commonly, miosis, ptosis, and cheek edema. Although both migraine and cluster headaches may respond to treatment with ergotamine, they are generally considered to be distinct entities.

444.   The answer is E. *(Adams, ed 4. pp 37-53.)* Diffuse hyperreflexia of an arm or leg indicates upper motor neuron dysfunction at a segmental level above that which supplies the involved limbs. Although weakness can be present with both upper and lower motor neuron lesions, marked muscle atrophy indicates axonal dysfunction in the lower motor neurons that innervate the limb's muscles. Thus, the combination of limb hyperreflexia and significant muscle atrophy can be seen only in conditions causing both upper and lower motor neuron dysfunction of multiple segments. Amyotrophic lateral sclerosis is such a condition. Both brachial plexus neuropathy and cervical radiculopathy affect only the lower motor neurons, causing segmental weakness, atrophy, and depressed or absent tendon reflexes. Cerebral infarction and multiple sclerosis usually disrupt the corticospinal tracts unilaterally or bilaterally, causing weakness and spastic hyperreflexia with little or no atrophy.

445.   The answer is C. *(Adams, ed 4. pp 821-824, 837-840.)* Wernicke's disease, as exemplified in the patient presented in the question, is characterized by ocular disturbances consisting of (1) weakness or paralysis of external recti, (2) nystagmus, and (3) paralysis of conjugate gaze. Ataxia and mental confusion complete the clinical picture. Many affected patients also demonstrate a peripheral poly-neuropathy. Korsakoff's psychosis, known also as amnestic-confabulatory psycho-sis, is not a separate disease but a variably present psychic component of Wernicke's disease involving impairment of retentive memory and learning ability. When both neurologic and psychic elements of the disease are present, it is known as Wernicke-Korsakoff syndrome. Marchiafava-Bignami disease, which is seen chiefly in Italian men who are heavy wine drinkers, is associated with bilateral demyelination of the corpus callosum; clinically, this disease is characterized by (1) emotional disorders, (2) loss of mental faculties, (3) convulsions, and (4) a variety of motor disabilities. Alcoholic cerebellar degeneration occurs twice as frequently as Wernicke's disease. It is characterized by a wide-based gait, truncal instability, and limb ataxia usually limited to the legs.

446.   The answer is B. *(Adams, ed 4. pp 276-277.)* The condition of brain death indicates that a patient, despite continued cardiac function, is dead based on neuro-logic criteria and testing. This type of testing is used when a severely brain-damaged patient, artificially maintained on a ventilator, shows no sign of brain function. Diagnosis of brain death requires demonstration of the following: (1) absence of all cerebral functions, i.e., deep coma, lack of convulsions, no decerebrate or decorti-cate posturing; (2) absence of all brainstem functions, i.e., absence of cranial nerve reflexes (pupillary, corneal, oculocephalic, oculovestibular, oropharyngeal) and presence of absolute apnea; and (3) irreversibility of the clinical state. The last criterion is generally determined by repeat clinical testing at least 6 h after the first examination and by obtaining tests for sedative-hypnotic drug overdose in the appropriate clinical setting.

447. The answer is E (all). *(Adams, ed 4. pp 314–316.)* The chief and usually first symptom of the narcolepsy syndrome is excessive daytime sleepiness. A patient will have frequent attacks (two to six per day) of irresistible drowsiness that come on following meals or periods of inactivity. Short periods of sleep follow, rarely lasting for more than 15 min. At the end of this time, patients awake feeling refreshed. Attacks of cataplexy are commonly present in patients with narcolepsy. This disorder is a sudden paralysis or loss of muscle tone brought on by strong emotion such as laughter or anger. Although the patient may fall to the ground, consciousness is always preserved. Also commonly seen with narcolepsy are vivid, often terrifying hallucinations on falling asleep (hypnagogic hallucinations) and brief loss of voluntary movements that just precede or follow sleep (sleep paralysis). It has been shown that a basic defect in sleep regulation exists in these patients. Characteristically, normal persons on falling asleep will have 1 to 2 h of non-REM sleep before they enter their first REM period; during the night they will then alternate between non-REM and REM periods. Patients with narcolepsy fall into REM sleep very quickly. This "short-latency," or early-onset, REM sleep can be recorded by polygraphic recordings in qualified sleep laboratories.

448. The answer is D (4). *(Adams, ed 4. pp 827–830, 1028–1034, 1042–1051.)* The term *polyneuropathy* indicates a diffuse and symmetrical dysfunction of the peripheral nerves, most commonly in the limbs but also commonly involving cranial nerves and nerves to the trunk. Clinical features often include distal sensory loss, distal and sometimes proximal weakness, reflex loss, and autonomic changes. There are two major pathologic processes that can affect the peripheral nerves in polyneuropathy. In segmental demyelination, there is a focal degeneration of myelin sheaths with sparing of axons. In axonal degeneration, neuronal disease results in degeneration of axon cylinders along with their myelin. Most polyneuropathies can be classified based on clinical presentation, electrodiagnostic studies (EMG and nerve conduction studies), and sural nerve biopsy. Axonal degeneration is the pathologic substate of most metabolic and toxic neuropathies with a subacute or chronic course. Metabolic etiologies include diabetes mellitus, the deficiency state associated with alcoholism, occult carcinoma, uremia, and vitamin B_{12} deficiency. Toxic etiologies include various drugs (isoniazid, hydralazine, nitrofurantoin, vincristine), heavy metals (arsenic, lead), and industrial solvents (*n*-hexane). Chronic polyneuropathies with primarily segmental demyelination are much less common. Chronic inflammatory polyradiculoneuropathy (CIP) shows many of the features of the Guillain-Barré syndrome (acute inflammatory polyradiculoneuropathy), namely, a symmetrical motor-sensory neuropathy, segmental demyelination on electrodiagnostic and pathologic studies, and cytoalbuminologic dissociation of the CSF. It differs from Guillain-Barré syndrome in that its course is either steadily progressive over many months or relapsing after spontaneous or drug-induced remissions.

449.   The answer is B (1, 3). *(Adams, ed 4. pp 572–573, 580–581, 1081–1083.)* Facial palsy as an isolated presenting complaint is common in clinical medicine. It generally indicates peripheral (infranuclear) facial nerve dysfunction and can be recognized by the following ipsilateral signs: inability to wrinkle the forehead, weakness of eye closure, decreased nasolabial fold, drooping of the mouth, and inability to smile. Although idiopathic facial (Bell's) palsy is the most common disease of the facial nerve, less common etiologies should be considered, especially in the presence of bilateral involvement. Sarcoidosis can affect both the peripheral and central nervous system, and the uveoparotid syndrome of sarcoidosis can cause a bilateral facial palsy. More recently, Lyme disease, a tick-borne spirochete infection, has surfaced as a major cause of peripheral facial nerve disease. The most common neurologic complications of Lyme disease are meningitis, cranial neuropathies (especially facial nerve), and radiculopathies, although numerous other central and peripheral manifestations have been reported.

450.   The answer is B (1, 3). *(Adams, ed 4. pp 649–651.)* TIAs are due to athero-sclerotic vascular disease and are reversible neurologic deficits that last no more than 24 h and usually less than 30 min. In one study, the 5-year cumulative rate of cerebral infarction was 22.7 percent and, for those with carotid lesions, the rate of myocardial infarction was 21 percent. There are no characteristics that distinguish those patients with TIAs who will go on to stroke from those who will not. TIAs of the carotid system typically result in either ipsilateral monocular blindness or contralateral sensorimotor disturbances; they do not occur simultaneously. TIAs of the vertebrobasilar system are characterized by various combinations of the following symptoms: dysarthria, bifacial numbness, dizziness, diplopia, and weakness or numbness of one or both sides of the body.

451.   The answer is C (2, 4). *(Adams, ed 4. pp 709–710.)* Epilepsy occurs in 5 percent of patients with closed-head injuries and only in those who sustain a contusion or laceration of the cerebral cortex. The seizures are either focal or generalized and only rarely are they of the petit mal variety. The timing of posttraumatic seizures varies; approximately half of patients who develop epilepsy will have their first attack within 6 months of injury. These seizures tend to decrease in frequency with time and up to 30 percent of patients will stop having them. Patients who have their first attack within a week of injury are more likely to have a complete remission than those patients whose first attack occurs over a year after trauma.

452.   The answer is B (1, 3). *(Adams, ed 4. pp 509–510.)* Pseudotumor cerebri is a syndrome of unknown origin characterized by extreme elevations of CSF pressure, typically from 250 to 450 mmH$_2$O. Patients present complaining of headache, blurred vision, and dizziness. The neurologic examination is significant for papilledema and, rarely, for an abducens palsy or nystagmus. Visual field testing shows enlargement of the blind spots along with peripheral constriction. Otherwise, the examination is usually unremarkable, with preserved mentation and alertness. The only severe consequence of this entity is visual loss in patients who do not respond to either repeated lumbar punctures or lumbar thecoperitoneal shunting. Therapy with steroids or oral hyperosmotic agents may be of benefit but is controversial.

453. The answer is A (1, 2, 3). *(Adams, ed 4. pp 932-935.)* Huntington's chorea is an autosomal dominant disorder characterized by choreoathetosis and dementia. It is believed to be due to an increased sensitivity of striatal receptors to dopamine. Both pathologically and on CT scan a bilateral wasting of the head of the caudate nucleus and putamen is seen. Patients present with disturbances in mood, poor self-control, changes in personality, a gradual fall in intellect, and choreoathetosis. The movement disorder may precede, follow, or occur at the same time as the mental symptoms. Huntington's chorea runs a progressive course, with death occurring an average of 15 years after onset; many of these patients are found to have chronic subdural hematomas related to frequent bouts of head trauma.

454. The answer is A (1, 2, 3). *(Adams, ed 4. p 164.)* Low back pain with radicular pain radiating down the leg (sciatica) is usually due to a herniated intervertebral disk compressing one of the lumbosacral roots, most commonly L5 or S1. The clinical history and neurologic examination can often indicate the specific nerve root involved. With lesions of the first sacral (S1) root, pain typically occurs in the midgluteal region, posterior thigh and calf, and outer plantar surface of the foot. Paresthesias and sensory loss occur in the posterior ankle, lateral foot, and outer (fourth and fifth) toes. Muscle weakness, if present, involves the flexors of the foot and toes and is manifested as difficulty walking on the toes. Most patients with an S1 radiculopathy have a diminished or absent ankle (Achilles) reflex.

455. The answer is E (all). *(Adams, ed 4. pp 381-383.)* Aphasia is a cerebral disturbance in language brought on most commonly by vascular lesions in the left, or dominant, perisylvian region. Broca's aphasia—also known as motor, expressive, or nonfluent aphasia—is characterized by markedly decreased word output and slow, disordered speech despite the normal functioning of the muscles of articulation. Repetition of spoken language is always abnormal, while most patients have a correspondingly severe impairment in writing. Comprehension of spoken and written language, impaired in Wernicke's aphasia, is generally preserved in Broca's aphasia. Lesions causing Broca's aphasia usually involve the left inferior frontal gyrus and frontoparietal operculum and adjacent cerebrum. Because of extension of the lesion and surrounding edema to adjacent frontal cortex, there is a frequently associated paresis of the right face and arm.

456. The answer is B (1, 3). *(Adams, ed 4. pp 1069, 1093.)* Knowledge of the anatomic relationships within the brachial plexus is essential for proper localization of a deficit causing weakness in an upper limb. The brachial plexus is formed from cervical roots 5, 6, 7, and 8 and the first thoracic root. Roots C5 and C6 merge into the upper trunk, root C7 forms the middle trunk, and roots C8 and T1 merge into the lower trunk. Key muscles affected by upper trunk lesions include serratus anterior, supraspinatus, infraspinatus, deltoid, biceps, and brachioradialis.

457. The answer is D (4). *(Adams, ed 4. pp 756–763.)* Multiple sclerosis is a chronic demyelinating disease of the central nervous system characterized by recurrent episodes or attacks of neurologic dysfunction related to multifocal disease of the optic nerves, spinal cord, and brain. Following attacks, neurologic dysfunction typically improves or remits over days to weeks, with new attacks or exacerbations sometimes occurring years later. Classic findings include weakness, impaired vision, nystagmus, dysarthria, impaired sensation, bladder dysfunction, and paraparesis. Ataxia is common and may be due to a cerebellar lesion, a lesion of the posterior columns (sensory ataxia), or both. Seizures occur in only 2 to 3 percent of patients with multiple sclerosis. Peripheral nerve involvement is extremely rare and can never be considered as a presenting sign of this disease.

458. The answer is C (2, 4). *(Adams, ed 4. pp 549, 1159–1160.)* Carcinomatous cerebellar degeneration is a rare but well-recognized nonmetastatic effect of neoplasia, most commonly associated with lung and ovarian carcinoma and lymphoma. The cerebellar signs, which precede the recognition of a neoplasm in half the cases, include gait and limb ataxia, dysarthria, and nystagmus. The disease is felt to be due to autoimmune factors, based on the finding of anti-Purkinje cell antibodies in patient sera. The Lambert-Eaton myasthenic syndrome is marked by weakness and fatigability primarily in the limb girdle and trunk muscles. Ocular and bulbar symptoms are less common. Other features are diminished deep tendon reflexes, dry mouth, and aching pain. As with cerebellar degeneration, neurologic symptoms may precede discovery of the tumor (usually oat cell carcinoma of the lung) by months or years. Studies have indicated a defect in the release of acetylcholine quanta from the nerve terminal at the neuromuscular junction. Electrodiagnostic studies (repetitive nerve stimulation at rapid rates) should reveal a characteristic incrementing response.

459–463. The answers are: 459-B, 460-A, 461-E, 462-C, 463-D. *(Adams, ed 4. pp 524–536.)* Glioblastoma multiforme accounts for 20 percent of all intracranial tumors and is highly malignant. While predominantly cerebral in location, tumors may be found in the cerebellum, brainstem, or spinal cord. Malignant cells may form distant foci on spinal roots or cause a meningeal gliomatosis; extraneural metastases are very rare. About 50 percent are bilateral or occur in more than one lobe of a hemisphere. The prognosis is poor as less than a fifth of all patients survive for 1 year after onset of symptoms.

An astrocytoma may occur anywhere in the brain or spinal cord. It is slowly growing and infiltrative and has a tendency to form large cavities (pseudocysts).

Calcium may be deposited in the tumor and seen on CT scan. Half of patients present with focal or generalized seizures. Seizures, headaches, and mental symptoms may be present for many years before diagnosis. In cases of cerebral astrocytoma, the average survival after the first symptom is 5 years; for cerebellar tumors, it is 7 years.

A meningioma is a benign tumor that is always sharply demarcated from brain tissue and is slowly growing. The most common sites are the sylvian region, superior parasagittal surface of frontal and parietal lobes, olfactory groove, lesser wing of the sphenoid bone, tuberculum sellae, superior surface of the cerebellum, cerebellopontine angle, and spinal canal. Surgical excision affords a permanent cure.

Medulloblastoma, primarily a childhood tumor, arises in the posterior part of the cerebellar vermis and neuroepithelial roof of the fourth ventricle. It is well demarcated from the adjacent brain tissue. Typically, patients present complaining of repeated vomiting and morning headache, followed by a stumbling gait, frequent falls, and a squint. Therapy with surgery, radiation of the neuraxis, and chemotherapy yields a 5-year survival in more than two-thirds of cases.

Hemangioblastoma of the cerebellum is characterized by dizziness, ataxia of gait, and signs and symptoms of increased intracranial pressure. Polycythemia may result from elaboration of an erythropoietic factor from the tumor. When seen with von Hippel-Lindau disease, the hemangioblastoma is associated with retinal angiomatoses and renal cysts. Surgical removal, when complete, is generally curative as regards the tumor.

464–467. The answers are: 464-E, 465-C, 466-D, 467-B. *(Adams, ed 4. pp 507–508, 609–610, 923–931.)* Alzheimer's disease is the most common degenerative disease of the brain, usually occurring in patients in their late fifties and older. The disease is highlighted by progressive dementia, which begins with memory deficits and personality changes and progresses to involve disorders of cerebral function, including aphasias, agnosias, and apraxias. Pathologic changes in the cerebral cortex include neuritic (senile) plaques, neurofibrillary tangles within nerve cells, and granulovacuolar degeneration of neurons.

Multi-infarct, or arteriosclerotic, dementia indicates intellectual impairment as a result of multiple cerebral strokes. Patients usually have a stuttering course with a temporal profile of distinct neurologic events (indicating strokes) associated with progression of dementia. Multiple infarcts may also produce a picture of pseudobulbar palsy (i.e., slurred speech, dysphagia, and emotional overflow).

Creutzfeldt-Jakob disease, also known as subacute spongiform encephalopathy, is a nervous system disease marked by a rapidly progressive dementia, diffuse myoclonic jerks, and cerebellar ataxia. Many patients have a distinctive EEG pattern consisting of generalized sharp wave complexes recurring at a rate of one per second. Gibbs has shown that the disease can be transmitted to primates by injecting them with diseased brain tissue. Iatrogenic disease has also occurred in patients who received growth hormone prepared from pooled cadaveric pituitary glands.

Normal pressure hydrocephalus (NPH) is thought to be due to nonprogressive meningeal and ependymal diseases and is characterized by enlarged ventricles with minimal or no brain atrophy. Patients with NPH manifest a clinical triad of progressive gait disorder, urinary incontinence, and dementia. CT scanning or radionuclide cisternography can usually verify the diagnosis of NPH, which may be cured by a ventricular shunt procedure.

468-471.   The answers are: 468-B, 469-C, 470-A, 471-B. *(Adams, ed 4. pp 251-254.)* Typical absence, or petit mal, seizure is the most characteristic epilepsy of childhood, with onset usually between age 4 and the early teens. Attacks, which may occur as frequently as several hundred in a day, consist of sudden interruptions of consciousness. The child stares, stops talking or responding, often displays eye fluttering, and commonly shows automatisms such as lip smacking and fumbling movements of the fingers. Attacks end in 2 to 10 s with the patient fully alert and able to resume activities. The characteristic EEG abnormality associated with attacks is three-per-second spike and wave activity.

Complex partial seizures, also known as psychomotor seizures, are characterized by complex auras with psychic experiences and periods of impaired consciousness with altered motor behavior. Common psychic experiences include illusions, visual or auditory hallucinations, feelings of familiarity (déjà vu) or strangeness (jamais vu), and fear or anxiety. Motor components include automatisms (e.g., lip smacking) and so-called automatic behavior (walking around in a daze, undressing in public). The brain lesion is usually in the temporal lobe, less commonly in the frontal lobe, and is often manifest as a focal epileptiform abnormality on EEG. Postictal confusion or drowsiness is the rule.

472-475.   The answers are: 472-C, 473-B, 474-C, 475-A. *(Adams, ed 4. pp 1035-1039, 1150-1152.)* Guillain-Barré syndrome, also known as acute inflammatory polyradiculoneuropathy, is an acute demyelinating polyneuropathy characterized by diffuse limb weakness that progresses to a maximum deficit over 2 to 3 weeks. As the syndrome develops, typical findings include proximal and distal limb weakness, ophthalmoplegias with facial weakness, areflexia, and, frequently, respiratory insufficiency. The CSF shows an elevated protein with normal white cell count (albuminocytologic dissociation) and the EMG/nerve conduction study indicates a demyelinating neuropathy.

Myasthenia gravis is a disease of the neuromuscular junction that results in fluctuating and sometimes persistent weakness of ocular, bulbar, limb, and respiratory muscles. More than 90 percent of patients develop extraocular palsies or ptosis, and 80 percent develop some weakness of the muscles of facial expression, mastication, swallowing, or speech. Diaphragmatic muscle weakness can lead to respiratory insufficiency. Sensory function and deep tendon reflexes are preserved. Weakened muscles usually improve dramatically upon administration of anticholinesterase drugs such as edrophonium (Tensilon).

Dermatology

DIRECTIONS: Each question below contains five suggested responses. Select the **one best** response to each question.

476. The skin cancer most likely to appear as a painless, pearly, ulcerated nodule with overlying telangiectasias is

(A) bowenoid actinic keratosis
(B) basal cell carcinoma
(C) squamous cell carcinoma
(D) superficial spreading melanoma
(E) glomus tumor

477. All the following skin tumors are caused by human papillomavirus (HPV) EXCEPT

(A) bowenoid papulosis of the penis
(B) condyloma accuminatum
(C) molluscum contagiosum
(D) plantar warts
(E) verruca plana (flat warts)

478. Pyoderma gangrenosum is associated with all the following EXCEPT

(A) inflammatory bowel disease
(B) vasculitis
(C) primary biliary cirrhosis
(D) trauma
(E) lack of response to antibiotic therapy

479. A 20-year-old woman is complaining of several days of low-grade fever, malaise, and mild conjunctivitis. Soon after the onset of fever, she developed a rash along with swelling of the joints of fingers, wrists, and knees in a symmetric fashion. The rash consists of discrete pink macules, which began on her face and extended to her trunk. She is also noted to have small red spots on her palate. Her arthritis is a complication of which of the following?

(A) Toxic shock syndrome
(B) Porphyria cutanea tarda
(C) Reiter's syndrome
(D) Rubella
(E) Gonococcal bacteremia

480. Increased risk factors for the development of cutaneous melanoma include all the following EXCEPT

(A) a changing nevus
(B) a large, congenital melanocytic nevus
(C) multiple dysplastic nevi
(D) a family history of melanoma
(E) type IV heavily pigmented skin

481. A 17-year-old girl noted a 2-cm, annular, pink, scaly lesion on her thigh. In the next two weeks she developed several smaller, oval, pink lesions with a fine collarette of scale. They seem to run in the body folds and mainly involve the trunk, although a few are on the upper arms and thighs. There is no adenopathy and no oral lesions. The most likely diagnosis is

(A) tinea versicolor
(B) psoriasis
(C) lichen planus
(D) pityriasis rosea
(E) secondary syphilis

482. All the following statements about aphthous stomatitis (canker sores) are correct EXCEPT

(A) the lesions occur singly or in groups and usually heal in 10 to 14 days
(B) the lesions are often seen in Behçet's syndrome
(C) coxsackievirus is frequently cultured from the lesions
(D) aphthous stomatitis can be associated with Crohn's disease
(E) at least 20 percent of the general population suffer the pain and discomfort of these outbreaks

483. Generalized exfoliative dermatitis is caused by which of the following disorders?

(A) Erythema multiforme
(B) Pemphigus vulgaris
(C) Mycosis fungoides
(D) Angiokeratoma corporis diffusum
(E) Atrophoderma of Pasini and Pierini

484. All the following mucocutaneous findings are associated with HIV infection EXCEPT

(A) morbilliform exanthem
(B) oral hairy leukoplakia
(C) dermatitis herpetiformis
(D) bacillary (or epithelioid) angiomatosis
(E) severe seborrheic dermatitis

485. A 20-year-old white man has noted an uneven tan on his upper back and chest. On examination he has many circular, lighter macules with a barely visible scale that coalesce into larger areas. The best test procedure you would use to establish the diagnosis is

(A) punch biopsy
(B) potassium hydroxide (KOH) microscopic examination
(C) a dermatophyte test medium (DTM) culture for fungus
(D) a serologic test for syphilis
(E) Tzanck smear

486. Herpes zoster (shingles) is characterized by all the following statements EXCEPT that it

(A) is caused by varicella virus
(B) typically produces grouped vesicles that may ulcerate and scar
(C) has a rate of recurrence of over 20 percent
(D) is not contagious for people who have had chickenpox
(E) has a significant association with malignant lymphoma

487. A 39-year-old woman has had nonhealing painful erosions in her mouth for the past year. She now observes rapidly spreading blisters on her chest and erosions on her scalp; the lesions are flaccid and red at the base. A biopsy report notes acantholysis of the prickle cells and deposition of IgG and complement in the intercellular spaces of the epidermis. Which of the following statements best summarizes both this woman's disorder and the appropriate treatment?

(A) She has bullous pemphigoid and should be treated with potent topical steroids applied every 2 to 3 h
(B) She has bullous erythema multiforme and should be treated with 6-mercaptopurine or methotrexate
(C) She has a disease that is fatal unless treated with oral prednisone, often requiring 100 mg or more daily
(D) She has cutaneous lupus erythematosus and should receive oral hydroxychloroquine, 400 mg a day
(E) She has bullous impetigo and needs oral penicillinase-resistant antibiotics for 7 to 10 days

488. Psoriasis is characterized by all the following statements EXCEPT

(A) it affects about 2 percent of the population
(B) lesions rarely occur on the scalp, but when they do they cause hair loss
(C) it consists of distinct red scaling papules or plaques on extensor surfaces
(D) the nails may have onycholysis, pits, and splinter hemorrhages
(E) an associated arthritis may occur

489. Generalized exfoliative dermatitis (erythroderma) is characterized by all the following statements EXCEPT that it

(A) can occur in a patient with psoriasis following the withdrawal of systemic steroids
(B) occurs in association with a T-cell lymphoma
(C) can occur in children with atopic dermatitis
(D) can occur in pityriasis rubra pilaris—a rare papulosquamous disease
(E) is an acute bullous condition that will resolve spontaneously

490. A young woman has recurrent episodes, lasting 1 to 2 weeks, of very painful ulcers scattered over the labial and buccal mucosa and occasionally on the pharynx. No blisters appear. Her lesions have no apparent association with stress, fever, or menses. The oval ulcers are 1 to 2 mm in size with a gray base and red border. The most likely diagnosis is

(A) herpes simplex
(B) herpes zoster
(C) aphthous stomatitis
(D) contact dermatitis
(E) desquamative gingivitis

491. A 28-year-old woman who is 3 months post partum notes a distressing loss of scalp hair. The patient takes no medications and says that she feels well. A meticulous physical examination is unremarkable; the scalp and hair appear normal, and there are no bald spots. However, several hairs were easily plucked out and had a small white bulb at the tip. The most likely cause of hair loss is

(A) lupus erythematosus
(B) postpartum telogen effluvium
(C) hypervitaminosis due to vitamin supplementation during pregnancy
(D) trichotillomania
(E) alopecia areata

492. The combination of psoralens and long ultraviolet light (PUVA) is effective in all the following diseases EXCEPT

(A) psoriasis
(B) vitiligo
(C) eczema
(D) mycosis fungoides
(E) porphyria cutanea tarda

493. Diabetes mellitus is associated with all the following cutaneous signs EXCEPT

(A) bacterial and fungal infections of the skin
(B) necrobiosis lipoidica diabeticorum (NLD)
(C) lipoatrophy
(D) brown atrophic macules on the pretibial surface
(E) lichen planus

494. Generalized pruritus without diagnostic skin lesions occurs in all the following conditions EXCEPT

(A) hyperthyroidism
(B) polycythemia vera
(C) carcinoid syndrome
(D) secondary syphilis
(E) pregnancy

495. All the following are cutaneous signs of internal disease EXCEPT

(A) necrobiosis lipoidica diabeticorum (NLD)
(B) lichen planus
(C) Paget's disease of the breast
(D) Kaposi's sarcoma
(E) eruptive xanthomas

496. An ill patient presents with a raised, nonblanching, violaceous, and widespread rash (palpable purpura). You must consider all the following diagnoses EXCEPT

(A) allergic vasculitis
(B) staphylococcal septicemia
(C) thrombocytopenia
(D) gonococcemia
(E) meningococcemia

DIRECTIONS: Each question below contains four suggested responses of which
one or more is correct. Select

A	if	**1, 2, and 3**	are correct
B	if	**1 and 3**	are correct
C	if	**2 and 4**	are correct
D	if	**4**	is correct
E	if	**1, 2, 3, and 4**	are correct

497. Skin signs of internal malignancy include

(1) migratory thrombophlebitis
(2) ichthyosis
(3) hypertrichosis lanuginosa
(4) acanthosis nigricans

498. Nail pitting is associated with which of the following skin diseases?

(1) Scleroderma
(2) Psoriasis
(3) Lichen planus
(4) Alopecia areata

499. Lesions associated with Reiter's syndrome include

(1) painless oral ulcers
(2) circinate balanitis
(3) keratoderma blenorrhagica
(4) granuloma annulare

500. A 65-year-old man with a history of rheumatoid arthritis treated with an arsenical compound many years ago is now noted to have a lesion on the volar aspect of his right arm. It is a sharply demarcated, hyperkeratotic, fissured, brownish-red plaque that has extended gradually over the past few years. Which of the following should be included in this man's therapy?

(1) Surgical excision of the lesion
(2) Systemic chemotherapy
(3) Examinations to detect visceral neoplasia
(4) Psoralen photochemotherapy (PUVA)

Dermatology

Answers

476.   The answer is B. *(Fitzpatrick, ed 3. pp 760–762.)* The question presents the classic description of a basal cell carcinoma. Bowenoid actinic keratosis appears as a keratotic red macule. Squamous cell cancers are the most easily confused with basal cell cancers, but are usually duller with a hyperkeratotic center. Superficial spreading melanomas are normally larger than 1 cm and irregular in border with mixtures of brown/black and white, and occasionally blue or red colors. Glomus tumors occur near the nail as a painful encapsulated deep nodule.

477.   The answer is C. *(Cobb, J Am Acad Dermatol 22:547–566, 1990.)* Molluscum contagiosum is a pearly wartlike growth caused by a paravaccinia virus (poxvirus). Fifty different human papillomaviruses have been identified in the last few years by gene analysis. These double-stranded DNA viruses belong to the papovavirus group. Anogenital condyloma is usually due to types 6, 11, 16, 18, and 31. Importantly, types 16, 18, and 31 have been associated with premalignant and malignant lesions, such as bowenoid papulosis, cervical dysplasia, and carcinoma in women, and occasionally rectal carcinoma and penile carcinoma in males.

478.   The answer is C. *(Fitzpatrick, ed 3. pp 1328–1334.)* Pyoderma gangrenosum is a progressive ulcerative lesion with a necrotic base and ragged, overhanging borders. It usually begins as a painful, red nodule on the lower extremities. Because the ulceration involves the reticular layer of the dermis and subcutis, scarring occurs on healing. While it is associated with a variety of diseases, it may occur as an illness confined to the skin in 40 to 50 percent of cases. An interesting feature of pyoderma gangrenosum is the susceptibility of the lesion to occur at sites of trauma. The course of pyoderma gangrenosum is highly variable, although when associated with inflammatory bowel disease, it usually parallels the activity of the gastrointestinal dysfunction. Therapy usually involves high doses of corticosteroids.

479.   The answer is D. *(Wilson, ed 12. p 547.)* The patient presented has a classic case of arthritis secondary to rubella infection. The arthritis is most often seen in young adults although it does occur in children who have been vaccinated with the live, attenuated rubella vaccine. It typically begins soon after the onset of the rash and is self-limiting, usually lasting several weeks. Joint effusions are small and serologic tests are negative. It is a nondestructive arthritis even in patients who have years of recurrent attacks. Other viral infections associated with arthritis include hepatitis B, arboviruses, mumps, infectious mononucleosis, varicella, and adenoviruses.

480. The answer is E. *(Fitzpatrick, ed 3. pp 889-910, 947-954.)* All the listed choices are significant risk factors for cutaneous melanoma except dark skin. Melanoma is seen more frequently in fair-skinned persons and rarely occurs in blacks.

481. The answer is D. *(Fitzpatrick, ed 3. pp 982-990.)* The description of this papulosquamous disease is that of a classic case of pityriasis rosea. This disease occurs in about 10 percent of the population. It is usually seen in young adults on the trunk and proximal extremities. There is a rare inverse form that occurs in the distal extremities and occasionally the face. Pityriasis rosea is usually asymptomatic, although some patients have an early, mild, viral prodrome (malaise, low-grade fever, and so on) and itching may be significant. Drug eruptions, fungal infections, and secondary syphilis are often confused with this disease. Fungal infections are rarely as widespread and sudden in onset; potassium hydroxide (KOH) preparation will be positive. Syphilis usually has adenopathy, oral patches, and lesions on the palms and soles (a VDRL test will be strongly positive at this stage). Psoriasis, with its thick, scaly red plaques on extensor surfaces, should not cause confusion. A rare condition called guttate parapsoriasis should be suspected if the rash lasts more than 2 months, since pityriasis rosea usually clears spontaneously in 6 weeks.

482. The answer is C. *(Fitzpatrick, ed 3. pp 1173-1177. Wilson, ed 12. pp 246, 1277.)* Aphthous stomatitis is one of the most common afflictions of the mouth. Between 20 and 50 percent of people suffer occasional or recurrent outbreaks of aphthous ulcers. In one series 50 percent of health professionals questioned stated that they were victims of this disease. Viruses are not cultured from these lesions, although some of them may have a herpetic look to them. The coxsackie A-16 enterovirus does produce lesions on the lips and oral mucosa that are part of hand-foot-and-mouth disease. A brief prodrome of mild fever, malaise, and gastrointestinal discomfort is followed by the evolution of papulovesicular lesions in the mouth. It appears that aphthous stomatitis is most likely to result from immunologic damage to the mucous membranes. Whether this is a true autoimmune phenomenon or a secondary reaction to, for example, streptococcal antigens in the mouth, is not clear. In addition, a number of immunologic disorders feature aphthous stomatitis. These include Crohn's disease, ulcerative colitis, selective IgA deficiency, pernicious anemia, Behçet's syndrome, and Reiter's syndrome. Although a number of biologic response modifiers are being tried, the treatment remains largely symptomatic. Tetracycline suspension held in the mouth for a few minutes before swallowing has been successful for some patients. The lesions may be less painful and heal more rapidly if a steroid in a paste vehicle that will adhere to the oral mucosa is applied to the lesions.

483.   The answer is C. *(Wilson, ed 12. pp 312, 323.)* Mycosis fungoides, a lymphoma of the skin, can pass through several stages. The first is a diffuse erythroderma and exfoliative dermatitis. In the second phase, plaques develop, and in the third phase, tumors and nodules are found. Not everyone who has exfoliative dermatitis has mycosis fungoides. Exfoliative dermatitis has other causes such as psoriasis, drug reactions, seborrheic dermatitis, and pityriasis rubra pilaris. Erythema multiforme and pemphigus produce blisters. Angiokeratoma corporis diffusum (Fabry's disease) exhibits unusual capillaries in the skin, especially in the groin and eye, and may cause fatal renal disease. Atrophoderma of Pasini and Pierini is an atrophic disease virtually impossible to confuse with an erythroderma.

484.   The answer is C. *(Friedman-Kien, J Am Acad Dermatol 22:1306–1319, 1990.)* Dermatitis herpetiformis is an autoimmune chronic vesiculobullous disease of unknown etiology. A morbilliform exanthem similar to other viral exanthems is seen in the initial phases of HIV infection. Oral hairy leukoplakia, often confused with oral candidiasis because of its white color, is seen on the sides of the tongue. Its cause is thought to be Epstein-Barr virus. Bacillary, or epithelioid, angiomatosis is a red-blue vascular tumor caused by a bacillus similar to cat-scratch bacillus. This tumor may be easily confused with Kaposi's sarcoma—another vascular tumor commonly seen in AIDS patients (especially homosexual AIDS patients). The incidence of seborrheic dermatitis is three or four times as frequent in AIDS patients and is usually more severe than that seen in the general population. This may be due to an increase in the yeast *Pityrosporum ovale*, thought to be related to seborrheic dermatitis. Psoriasis may also be worse in patients with AIDS. Many other skin infections are common and more severe in AIDS patients (e.g., warts, molluscum contagiosum, and candidiasis).

485.   The answer is B. *(Fitzpatrick, ed 3. pp 2197–2200.)* The diagnosis is tinea versicolor, which can be confirmed by a KOH microscopic examination. Routine fungal cultures will not grow this yeast. A Wood's light examination will often show a green fluorescence, but it may be negative if the patient has recently showered. A Tzanck smear is used on blisters to detect herpes infections.

486.   The answer is C. *(Wilson, ed 12. pp 686–689.)* Most patients who have herpes zoster (shingles) are basically healthy and remain so. However, the disease occurs in 25 percent of patients who have lymphoma, Hodgkin's disease in particular. An affliction chiefly of adulthood, shingles arises from endogenous varicella virus that has lain dormant since the time of its original manifestation as chickenpox. Thus shingles—unlike chickenpox, which is caused by the same virus—is acquired not exogenously but from within. Children who have not been exposed to varicella-herpes zoster virus, when exposed to shingles, can develop chickenpox. There have been only occasional reports suggesting that shingles is directly transmittable and produces shingles in close contacts. Unlike herpes simplex, herpes zoster rarely recurs.

487. The answer is C. *(Wilson, ed 12. pp 318–319.)* The patient discussed in the question has an advanced stage of pemphigus vulgaris, a disease that is fatal unless properly treated with prednisone. The drug should be given orally, 100 mg daily or more. When affected patients have improved, the dose can be lowered and azathioprine (Imuran), gold, or methotrexate can be added to minimize the need for oral steroids. However, low-dose steroids or immunosuppressive agents early in the course of pemphigus are often unavailing. Approximately 30 percent of patients having this disease die from complications of treatment; of the survivors, many eventually dispense with medication entirely and lead normal lives.

488. The answer is B. *(Wilson, ed 12. p 309.)* Psoriatic lesions occur quite frequently on the scalp as well as on the elbows, knees, and sacrum. The scalp lesions are sharply demarcated, as are those on the rest of the skin. These sharply demarcated margins differentiate psoriasis from seborrheic dermatitis, which also commonly affects the scalp. Since the scales may be anchored by hair, they may "heap up" so that localized accumulations are usually felt. In contrast, seborrheic dermatitis does not produce this degree of accumulation; instead, it produces a diffuse, scaly erythema. Hair loss does not usually occur in psoriasis unless the hair is removed by excessive scratching of the lesions. Diagnostic nail changes consisting of onycholysis and pits in the nail plate are often seen. Psoriatic arthritis develops in about 10 percent of patients. Perhaps 90 percent of patients with psoriatic arthritis will at some point exhibit nail lesions.

489. The answer is E. *(Wilson, ed 12. p 323.)* The course of exfoliative dermatitis is determined by its cause. In patients with generalized skin disease (e.g., psoriasis), the disease usually responds to appropriate therapy, whereas in systemic disease (e.g., lymphoma), the prognosis is relatively poor. Withdrawal of systemic steroids often results in a worsening of psoriasis and may trigger a pustular psoriasis or exfoliative erythroderma. Although pityriasis rubra pilaris is rare, it will often manifest as an exfoliative erythroderma. Exfoliative dermatitis may occur as a result of a drug reaction, as a manifestation of a generalized preexisting dermatitis, or in association with systemic disease, such as T-cell lymphoma (mycosis fungoides) or leukemia. Approximately 60 percent of affected patients recover in less than a year, 10 percent have a persistent problem that does not respond to treatment, and up to 30 percent die.

490. The answer is C. *(Wilson, ed 12. pp 246, 1456.)* The patient presented in the question probably has aphthous ulcers, lesions that frequently are misdiagnosed as herpes simplex. Herpes tends to cause a group of shallow, round ulcers, frequently beginning as blisters and having a red or yellowish color at the base. These lesions can recur but usually not as often as aphthae. The cause of aphthae is unknown; repeated cultures for viruses, mycoplasma, and other pathogens have been negative. Moreover, attempts to treat the lesions with antibiotics have been unsuccessful. Topical steroids, while not curative, may be palliative. Topical anesthetics may provide symptomatic relief.

491.   The answer is B. *(Fitzpatrick, ed 3. pp 640–641.)* In the patient presented in the question, the most probable cause of hair loss is normal postpartum telogen effluvium. In the first trimester of pregnancy, telogen hairs (resting hairs) constitute a normal 15 to 20 percent of all hair; later in pregnancy, the telogen hair count may drop to 10 percent. This means that many follicles that normally would have reached the end of their active (anagen) phase are still present at parturition. Telogen counts rise quickly in the postpartum period, sometimes reaching 30 to 40 percent of total hair. Telogen lasts approximately 3 months. At the end of this period, there is abnormally heavy shedding while a normal telogen-to-anagen hair ratio is reestablished. A patient who presents with hair loss should be carefully examined for circular bald spots that might indicate alopecia areata or trichotillomania. Trichotillomania, which is loss of hair from pulling, usually causes bald areas with short hairs remaining. Lupus erythematosus and hypervitaminosis can both cause alopecia, but there is no reason to suspect them in this patient. Discoid lupus causes a scarring alopecia.

492.   The answer is E. *(Wilson, ed 12. pp 342–343.)* Psoralens in conjunction with ultraviolet radiation (UV-A, 320 to 400 nm) are frequently employed in treating psoriasis. The combination (PUVA) also has been widely used in treating vitiligo, eczema, and mycosis fungoides. In the presence of psoralen, irradiation with UV-A results in the binding of psoralen to pyrimidine bases in DNA. Although this reaction leads to inhibition of DNA synthesis followed by cell death, recent studies have indicated that PUVA may exert its effect by suppression of the immune response and other effects on cell membranes. This treatment should only be given by experienced dermatologists. Patients who are candidates for this regimen are exposed to a measured dose of ultraviolet radiation following ingestion of the medication. Repeated (PUVA) treatments (two or three times a week) are required to produce disappearance of psoriatic lesions. Possible side effects of this and other types of photochemotherapy include premature aging, cataracts, and skin cancer. Porphyrias are made worse by UV-A.

493.   The answer is E. *(Wilson, ed 12. p 1756.)* Lichen planus is not associated with diabetes mellitus. Necrobiosis lipoidica diabeticorum and lipoatrophy are virtually pathognomonic signs. Atrophic brown macules, termed *diabetic dermopathy*, also are classic manifestations of diabetes. Cutaneous bacterial and fungal infections (especially *Candida albicans*) are seen more frequently with diabetes.

494.   The answer is D. *(Wilson, ed 12. pp 655–656, 1320, 1344.)* A number of conditions are characterized by a generalized pruritus in the absence of recognizable skin lesions. Hyperthyroidism, carcinoid syndrome, and pruritus of pregnancy often are associated with cholestasis, which may be overt; affected patients may manifest jaundice or merely an elevation of serum alkaline phosphatase and bile acids. Syphilis causes a plethora of skin lesions—notably macules or papules in secondary syphilis. Pruritus in the absence of skin lesions is extremely rare in patients who have syphilis.

495.   The answer is B. *(Fitzpatrick, ed 3. pp 967, 973, 1078–1085, 1730, 1931, 2077.)* Lichen planus is not a cutaneous sign of internal disease. Diabetes occurs in over 50 percent of patients with NLD. This presents with atrophic, yellowish areas on the skin. The dermatitic rash of Paget's disease of the breast and extramammary Paget's disease is associated with underlying apocrine (mammary) carcinoma. In Kaposi's sarcoma, violaceous tumors are seen in immunosuppressed patients, especially in homosexual patients with AIDS. Eruptive xanthomas (yellow papules with erythematous halos) are seen in diabetes and hypertriglyceridemia.

496.   The answer is C. *(Fitzpatrick, ed 3. pp 1300–1302, 1910–1912.)* Palpable purpura is one of the most important cutaneous signs of internal disease. Its infectious causes listed in this question are life-threatening and death may occur in a few hours. Gram stain smears of the lesions can often make the diagnosis. In a patient with fever and other signs of infection, one cannot wait for a biopsy diagnosis. Vasculitis is probably one of the most common causes of a palpable purpura. The lesions are palpable because of the inflammatory cell infiltrate. Clotting disorders do not cause palpable purpura.

497.   The answer is E (all). *(Wilson, ed 12. pp 322–338, 1023.)* When no obvious cause for migratory thrombophlebitis is present, especially when that phlebitis involves areas other than the pelvis, a physician should be suspicious about an underlying malignancy. Often the phlebitis can precede the clinical symptoms and signs of a malignancy by many months. Although carcinoma of the pancreas is the most common tumor with which it is associated, it is by no means the only one. It is unusual to find an operable lesion associated with this sign, so the prognostic significance of the association is grave. Pulmonary embolism is an all-too-common complication. In ichthyosis, the skin appears dry and the stratum corneum sheds rhomboidal scales. In the absence of a family history of this disorder, its development strongly suggests the possibility of an underlying lymphoma. Hodgkin's disease has been the most common malignancy associated with ichthyosis. The increased hair growth associated with the condition hypertrichosis lanuginosa is distinctive. The hair is extremely fine with a silky texture and lightly pigmented. Growth may occur on the trunk, arms, and legs, but the most common sites are the face and ears. Although it can be difficult to differentiate this proliferation of lanugo from the effects seen in women with disorders of male sex hormones, the more florid forms of this syndrome are easily recognized. The mechanisms for the production of the hair growth are unclear, but there is a strong association with cancer involving the breast, bladder, lung, gallbladder, colon, and rectum. Acanthosis nigricans appears as a velvety, brown raised area in the body folds, especially on the neck axillae and groin. It has a characteristic appearance on biopsy. Acanthosis nigricans is associated most often with gastrointestinal cancers. It usually appears in people over 40 years of age. Pseudoacanthosis nigricans *must* be ruled out. The cause of the benign "pseudo" forms can be obesity, endocrine abnormalities, and, rarely, drugs (e.g., nicotinamide). It may be confused with lichenification, such as that seen in atopic dermatitis.

498.   The answer is C (2, 4). *(Fitzpatrick, ed 3. pp 654–658.)* Pits are the most common lesion of psoriatic nails and actually represent psoriatic lesions located in the matrix of the nail bed. As the nail plate emerges from the proximal nail fold, the keratotic plug falls off and a pit is formed. The pits typically vary in size, shape, and depth. In alopecia areata, nail pits commonly form in traverse rows. Nail atrophy and dystrophy in lichen planus can be profound, but pits are not characteristically seen.

499.   The answer is A (1, 2, 3). *(Fitzpatrick, ed 3. pp 1874–1882.)* Reiter's syndrome is characterized by arthritis, urethritis, and conjunctivitis occurring predominantly in men between the ages of 15 and 35. Mucocutaneous lesions occur in the majority of patients. Keratoderma blenorrhagica begins as brownish-red macules that develop into hyperkeratotic papules, which may coalesce; these lesions occur mainly on the palms and soles, although any part of the body may be involved. Circinate balanitis occurs on the glans penis as dry, crusting plaques in circumcised men and as shallow, painless ulcers in those uncircumcised. The oral lesions are painless ulcers found on the tongue and hard palate. All lesions heal without scarring.

500.   The answer is B (1, 3). *(Fitzpatrick, ed 3. pp 739–740. Wilson, ed 12. pp 1633–1634.)* The patient described has Bowen's disease, or squamous cell carcinoma of the skin in situ. Arsenical exposure has been implicated as causative in many cases of this disease. While most lesions do not become invasive and only 2 percent metastasize, their importance lies in their association with gastrointestinal, genitourinary, and pulmonary carcinomas. The risk of an associated neoplasm is particularly high when Bowen's disease occurs on parts of the body not usually exposed to sunlight. The development of a visceral neoplasm may occur many years after the onset of the skin lesion, and examinations for visceral cancer, therefore, should be done at intervals. The lesions should be surgically excised or treated by various methods of local destruction.

Bibliography

Adams, RA, Victor M: *Principles of Neurology*, 4th ed. New York, McGraw-Hill, 1989.

Balow JE: Renal vasculitis. *Kidney Int* 27:954–964, 1985.

Bart KJ, et al: The current status of immunization principles: Recommendations for use and adverse reactions. *J Allergy Clin Immunol* 79:296–315, 1987.

Berk JE, Haubrich WS, Kalser MH, et al (eds): *Bockus Gastroenterology*, 4th ed. Philadelphia, WB Saunders, 1985.

Braunwald E (ed): *Heart Disease*, 3d ed. Philadelphia, WB Saunders, 1988.

Buckley RH: Immunodeficiency diseases. *JAMA* 258:2841–2850, 1987.

Cappell MS: The hepatobiliary manifestations of the acquired immunodeficiency syndrome. *Am J Gastroenterol* 86:1–15, 1991.

Centers for Disease Control: 1989 Sexually transmitted diseases treatment guidelines. *MMWR* 38 (S-8), 1989.

Chow AW, Jenesson PJ: Pharmacokinetics and safety of antimicrobial agents during pregnancy. *Rev Infect Dis* 7:287–313, 1985.

Cobb MW: Human papillomavirus infection. *J Am Acad Dermatol* 22:547–566, 1990.

Eastwood GL, Avunduck C: *Manual of Gastroenterology: Diagnosis and Therapy*. Boston, Little, Brown, 1988.

Felig P, Baxter JD, Broadus, AE, Frohman LA: *Endocrinology and Metabolism*, 2d ed. New York, McGraw-Hill, 1987.

Fink JN, de Shazo R: Immunologic aspects of granulomatous and interstitial lung disease. *JAMA* 258:2938–2944, 1989.

Fishman AP: *Pulmonary Diseases and Disorders*, 2d ed. New York, McGraw-Hill, 1988.

Fitzpatrick TB, Eisen A, Wolff K, et al: *Dermatology in General Medicine*, 3d ed. New York, McGraw-Hill, 1987.

Forrester JS, Diamond G, Chatterjee K, et al: Medical therapy of acute myocardial infarction by application of hemodynamic subsets. *N Engl J Med* 295:1356-1360, 1976.

Friedman-Kien AE: HIV disease, from discovery to management: The major role of the dermatologist. *J Am Acad Dermatol* 22:1306-1319, 1990.

Greenberger PA, Patterson R: Diagnosis and management of allergic broncholpulmonary aspergillosis. *Ann Allergy* 56:144-148, 1986.

Grieco MH, Meriney DK: *Immunodiagnosis for Clinicians: Interpretation of Immunoassays*. Chicago, Year Book Medical, 1983.

Gross NJ: Pulmonary effects of radiation therapy. *Ann Intern Med* 86:81-92, 1977.

Hanifin JM: Atopic dermatitis. *J Allergy Clin Immunol* 73:211-222, 1984.

Heffner JE, Miller KS, Sahn SA: Tracheostomy in the ICU, parts I and II. *Chest* 90:269-273, 430-435, 1986.

Holic MF: Vitamin D and the kidney. *Kidney Int* 32:912-929, 1987.

Hoshino PK, Gaasch WH: When to intervene in chronic aortic regurgitation. *Arch Intern Med* 146:349-352, 1986.

Houston MC: New insights and new approaches for the treatment of essential hypertension. *Am Heart J* 117:911-951, 1989.

Hurst JW, Schlant RC, Rackley CE, et al (eds): *The Heart*, 7th ed. New York, McGraw-Hill, 1990.

Levy MB, Fink JN: Hypersensitivity pneumonitis. *Ann Allergy* 54:167-171, 1985.

Mandel WJ: *Cardiac Arrhythmias: Their Mechanisms, Diagnosis and Management*, 2d ed. Philadelphia, JB Lippincott, 1987.

Mandell GL, Douglas RG Jr, Bennett JE: *Principles and Practice of Infectious Diseases*, 3d ed. New York, Churchill Livingstone, 1990.

Massry SG, Glassock RJ (eds): *Textbook of Nephrology*, 2d ed. Baltimore, Williams & Wilkins, 1989.

McCarty GA: *Arthritis and Allied Conditions*, 11th ed. Philadelphia, Lea & Febiger, 1989.

Med Lett Drugs Ther: Gonadorelin-synthetic LH-RH. 25:106, 1983.

Middleton E, et al (eds): *Allergy: Principles and Practice*, 3d ed. St. Louis, CV Mosby, 1988.

Murray JF, Nadel JA: *Textbook of Respiratory Medicine*. Philadelphia, WB Saunders, 1988.

O'Byrne PM, Dolovich J, Hargreave FE: State of art: Late asthmatic responses. *Am Rev Respir Dis* 136:740-741, 1987.

Patel HP, Anhalt GJ, Diaz LA: Bullous pemphigoid and pemphigus vulgaris. *Ann Allergy* 50:144-149, 1984.

Patterson R (ed): *Allergic Diseases: Diagnosis and Management*, 3d ed. Philadelphia, JB Lippincott, 1985.

Rackley CE: *Advances in Critical Care Cardiology*. Philadelphia, FA Davis, 1986.

Roitt IV, Brostoff J, Male DK: *Immunology*, 2d ed. St. Louis, CV Mosby, 1989.

Rose BD: *Clinical Physiology of Acid-Base and Electrolyte Disorders*, 3d ed. New York, McGraw-Hill, 1989.

Rose BD: *Pathophysiology of Renal Disease*, 2d ed. New York, McGraw-Hill, 1987.

Schiff L, Schiff ER: *Diseases of the Liver*, 6th ed. Philadelphia, JB Lippincott, 1987.

Sherlock S: *Diseases of the Liver and Biliary System*, 8th ed. Cambridge, MA, Blackwell Scientific, 1989.

Sleisenger MS, Fordtran JS: *Gastrointestinal Disease: Pathophysiology, Diagnosis, Management*, 4th ed. Philadelphia, WB Saunders, 1989.

Smolens P: The kidney in dysproteinemic states. *Am Kidney Fund Nephrol Lett*, vol 4, no 4, 1987.

Somberg JC, Muira D, Keefe DC: The treatment of ventricular rhythm disturbances. *Am Heart J* 111:1162-1176, 1986.

Spark RF, White RA, Hollowing DB: Impotence is not always psychogenic: New insights into hypothalamic-pituitary gonadal dysfunction. *JAMA* 243:730, 1980.

Stein JH, Hutton JJ, Kohler PD, et al: *Internal Medicine*, 3d ed. Boston, Little, Brown, 1990.

Stiehm ER, et al: Intravenous immunoglobulins as therapeutic agents. *Ann Intern Med* 107:367-382, 1987.

Stites DP, Stobo JD, Wells JV: *Basic and Clinical Immunology*, 6th ed. East Norwalk, CT, Appleton & Lange, 1987.

Strober W, James SP: The immunopathogenesis of gastrointestinal and hepatobiliary diseases. *JAMA* 258:2962-2969, 1987.

Wellens HF, Bar LW, Lie KI: The value of the electrocardiogram in the differential diagnosis of tachycardia with a widened QRS complex. *Am J Med* 64:27-33, 1978.

Williams WJ, et al (eds): *Hematology*, 4th ed. New York, McGraw-Hill, 1990.

Wilson JD, Braunwald E, Isselbacher KJ, et al (eds): *Harrison's Principles of Internal Medicine*, 12th ed. New York, McGraw-Hill, 1991.

Wyngaarden JB, Smith LH Jr (eds): *Cecil Textbook of Medicine*, 18th ed. Philadelphia, WB Saunders, 1988.

Zakim D, Boyer TD: *Hepatology: A Textbook of Liver Disease*, 2d ed. Philadelphia, WB Saunders, 1990.